UNDERSTANDING
the Basics for
Nursing Home
ADMINISTRATORS

A Guide to Success in Every
Department

A *TAB* Original
Houston, Texas

PO BOX 5156
Houston, TX 77325

Distributed by The Awesome Boss LLC

For ordering information or special discounts for bulk purchases, please contact The Awesome Boss LLC at PO Box 5156, Houston, TX, 77325, or betheawesomeboss@gmail.com.

Library of Congress Cataloging-In-Publication Data

Burningham, Tim.

Understanding the basics for nursing home administrators : a guide to success in every department / Tim Burningham — 1st ed.
p. ; cm.

Issued also as an ebook.

ISBN: 9781073332748

1.   Nursing Home Administration 2. Understanding Basics 3. Business 4. Health Care I. Title

Printed in the United States of America

First Edition

TAB 09 30 10 11 12 05 07

Also by Tim Burningham

The Wisdom Story: How to Create a High-Performing Company Culture and Transform Results

How Leaders Can Strengthen Their Organization's Culture

Be An Awesome Boss!: The Four C's Model to Leadership Success

Contents

Introduction...vi

Chapter 1: Industry Overview..1

Chapter 2: Creating Culture...6

Chapter 3: Common SNF Acronyms, Abbreviations, and Terms 12

Chapter 4: Housekeeping Department...32

Chapter 5: Laundry Department..37

Chapter 6: Maintenance Department 41

Chapter 7: Dietary Services..48

Chapter 8: Activities Department 55

Chapter 9: Social Services 62

Chapter 10: Medical Records..69

Chapter 11: Human Resources 75

Chapter 12: Payroll 82

Chapter 13: CNA Care 87

Chapter 14: Nursing Care...93

Chapter 15: Nursing Administration 100

Chapter 16: Nursing Systems..105

Chapter 17: Regulatory Basics 114

Chapter 18: CMS Star Rating 123

Chapter 19: Revenue and MDS..134

Chapter 20: Rehabilitation Services...142

Chapter 21: Business Office and Accounts Receivable 154

Chapter 22: Financial Management..161

Chapter 23: Accounts Payable 171

Chapter 24: Central Supply, Equipment, and Staffing 175

Chapter 25: Crucial Meetings 184

Chapter 26: Contracts and Vendors..192

Chapter 27: Marketing..197

Chapter 28: Admissions 205

Chapter 29: Customer Service 212

Chapter 30: The Basics..217

Acknowledgements..224

A Formula For Success... 225

About the Author 227

Introduction

Purpose

Being a licensed nursing home administrator (LNHA) is not easy. Unlike most professions, nursing home administrators are required to have a certain level of proficiency in a very wide range of disciplines and skills, such as providing a great dining experience, developing an engaging activity program, maintaining immaculate medical records, and ensuring that a large facility stays spotlessly clean—just to name a few. And, as if accumulating knowledge about every department within a skilled nursing facility (SNF) isn't enough, administrators are also expected to be savvy marketers, customer service gurus, human resources specialists, and caring and compassionate leaders. To put it simply, gaining the expertise one needs to be an effective administrator can be challenging.

The purpose of this book is to provide you with the essential knowledge you need about each SNF department, plus a few other critical topics. This book takes a simple, straightforward approach to arm you with information that will enable you to be a successful administrator and meet the myriad of challenges that come your way.

The Upside

Though it is not easy, being a nursing home administrator is a rewarding, exciting, and fast-paced career. Like few others, it allows you to meet and interact with a wide variety of people, help those in need, protect some of the most vulnerable in our society, and have an enormous influence on the lives of so many individuals. The bottom line is being an administrator is impactful.

Being an LNHA requires a tremendous amount of skill, dedication, and passion. It demands the very best from you. It pushes you to become a better leader and a better person.

The need for qualified and talented nursing home administrators in the United States will continue to grow rapidly over the next 10 to 15 years as the population ages and the number of individuals over 65 more than doubles. The time to step up and shine as a leader in the skilled nursing industry is now!

As a note, the terms resident, patient, and customer are used interchangeably throughout the book. Historically, the most common term used when referring to skilled nursing facility patrons had been residents, however with shorter stays in skilled nursing facilities, that has changed. Many short-term stay patrons, not wanting the perception that they are moving in or staying for an extended period of time, have resisted being called residents. Therefore, many SNFs have adopted the term patient or customer, especially when referring to short-term stay patrons. Since every facility is different in how they choose to call their patrons, I've taken liberty to use these terms interchangeably.

CHAPTER 1

Industry Overview

Introduction

Traditional nursing homes of the past, for the most part, have gone by the wayside. Rather than just being a place for a person to live until the day they die, SNFs are now tasked with focusing on shorter stays and moving patients quickly and safely to the next level of care (i.e. assisted living centers, senior housing, or home with home health care, etc.). In general, the lengths of stay for residents in SNFs are decreasing. Because of this, the patient population in a SNF now changes more frequently than in the past, with more frequent admissions and discharges.

Today's SNFs are expected to accommodate more complex and diverse patients. And this is to be done in a way that is more dignified and offers a higher quality of life to those they serve. Treatments and procedures that could once only be done at hospitals are now taking place at SNFs. For this reason, learning to handle a wider range of needs has become a primary challenge that facilities are striving to overcome.

New payment models have also challenged the traditional way of doing things. These payment models have created new ways to grow revenue and partner with other health care providers to coordinate and improve service across a continuum of care.

Unlike the past, SNFs today can be very different from one another. Many focus on specific niches in order to build census and stay competitive. For example, some facilities have a high population of long-term care residents, while others only accept short-term patients. Some emphasize rehabilitation care while others specialize in wound care and recovery. It is important for each facility to create a strategy that will best meet the needs of its unique community and lead to the facility's success.

Industry Metric

The most common financial metric in the skilled nursing industry is PPD, which means per patient day. This measurement enables the comparison of different facilities across a broad spectrum of areas within the business. The PPD metric essentially removes the variables and helps leaders determine how a facility is performing in comparison to others. It allows for an apples-to-apples comparison regardless of a facility's size, location, age, layout, etc. It also allows for comparisons between months, quarters, and years within the same facility.

There are two common types of PPD measurements used in the industry: hours PPD and dollars PPD. An example of hours PPD is the number of employee hours used in the dietary department per patient per day. An example of dollars PPD is the amount of money spent on food per patient per day.

A more comprehensive overview of PPDs including how to monitor and control your facility's PPDs will be covered in future chapters in this book. The PPD metric is often used to help evaluate the performance of a facility and of an administrator.

Interdisciplinary Team

Interdisciplinary team is a term you will hear often in the industry and throughout this book. So what is it? An interdisciplinary team is a group of individuals who work in different departments and have expertise in different disciplines. Its purpose is to take a wholistic approach when caring for residents.

In SNFs, it is important for facilities to take an interdisciplinary approach to setting up care plans, solving problems, and even providing care. Individuals with different expertise view a patient with a unique set of eyes and are trained to meet specific needs of the individual. Getting feedback and input from multiple disciplines enables a facility to make the best decisions and provide the best care for those they serve. An interdisciplinary approach to care, services, and even challenges within the facility is a wise approach.

Any group of individuals in a SNF from different departments can make up an interdisciplinary team. There are different situations, challenges, and discussions that call for different groups of people with different expertise—thus the makeup of the interdisciplinary team may vary for each situation. For example, a family member's question about a resident's diet may take an interdisciplinary discussion and response which may include the director of nursing, director of rehabilitation, and dietary manager but wouldn't necessarily include the activities director.

An Administrator's Skill Set

Probably the single most important trait of a successful licensed nursing home administrator (LNHA) is having great interpersonal skills. As an administrator, you work closely with a wide range of individuals of diverse backgrounds, experiences, socioeconomic statuses, and education levels. From housekeeping and laundry aides to physicians, therapists, and other health care professionals, administrators need to know how to work well with all different types of people.

On top of this, administrators will be caring for people who are facing some of the most difficult challenges and decisions of their life. Learning how to interact and work empathetically with family members and individuals who are often exhausted, confused, and stressed is key to an administrator's success.

In addition to outstanding interpersonal skills, LNHAs must also have training and knowledge in a wide range of disciplines such as nursing, rehabilitation, plant maintenance, housekeeping, and dietary services, to name just a few. Unfortunately, too many administrator-in-training programs do not adequately expose future administrators to all the areas of the facility they will one day be responsible for managing. But don't worry—this book is here to help!

Conclusion

The challenges of the industry are ever-changing, and this makes a career as an LNHA exciting and fast-paced. No two days are ever the same.

Since changes are so frequent, the industry needs leaders who are not only able to learn quickly, but who are also willing to adjust and be flexible in order to meet the needs of those they serve. Facilities that can develop the necessary clinical capabilities and skills to manage complex nursing needs and cater to a more diverse patient demographic will lead the way.

A career as an LNHA is extremely rewarding and allows you to have a tremendous impact on the lives of many people. As the U.S. population ages at an accelerated rate, the SNF industry, now more than ever, needs great leaders who are dedicated to the field and who want to make a real difference in the lives of others.

KEY TAKEAWAYS

- The industry is changing rapidly with shorter stays, a more diverse patient population, higher complexities of care, and different reimbursement systems.
- PPD means per patient day and is the most common measurement used in the industry. This measurement allows leaders to compare performance among very different facilities. A facility and an administrator are often judged on their ability to control and improve PPDs.
- LNHAs must be able to learn quickly and adjust even quicker to frequent changes in the industry in order to constantly meet the needs of those they serve.
- With the rapidity of our aging population, the demand for excellent leaders and administrators is growing quickly, making nursing home administration an attractive career choice.

CHAPTER 2

Creating Culture

Introduction

Above all else, the workplace culture you help create and maintain at your facility will have the biggest impact on its success. For this reason, we will start here before we dive into the different departments and aspects of a SNF.

Workplace culture is the shared beliefs, assumptions, and behaviors that exist within an organization. It includes the way people feel at work.

Workplace culture has huge ramifications on every aspect of your facility. It can help or hurt every problem and challenge you face. And now more than ever before, with nursing shortages increasing and the competition for talent steadily ramping up, the need to attract and retain the right team members is critical to your success. As an administrator, creating the right workplace culture should be your number-one priority. The right culture attracts the right people. The right people create the best clinical outcomes. And the best clinical outcomes go hand-in-hand with sustainable financial results.

In summary: culture → clinical → financial. Start by cultivating your workplace culture, and the rest will follow.

Great Workplace Culture = Best Clinical Outcomes = Excellent Financial Results

Where to Start

There are so many ways to influence your facility's culture. But first you must understand that as its leader, every action you take, everything you say, and the way you react and respond to different situations will have a significant impact. You cannot underestimate the influence you as an administrator personally has on the culture of your facility.

The building blocks of a strong culture are threefold:

1. **A mission.** What is your facility's mission or purpose? Why does your team wake up and come to work every day? What is the "why" behind it all? Helping everyone in your facility understand the "why," or the facility's mission, will go a long way in establishing the right culture.

2. **Core values.** Core values are often idealistic, and they give people standards to live by and aspire to. What do you represent and what is important to you? Ensuring all staff have a strong understanding of the facility's core values will positively impact its culture.

3. **Your vision.** What do you hope to accomplish long-term? Where do you see your facility in 10, 20, or even 50 years down the road? What positive contribution will the facility make to the community? This vision can help direct your path and inspire your people. Helping people understand what the facility is ultimately trying to become and accomplish—and how they can play a part in it—will help strengthen your culture.

Making sure everyone is not only aware of but also clearly understands the mission, core values, and vision for your facility is a great place to start in establishing the right culture. These building blocks will guide the decisions you make and influence how staff interact with customers and with one another.

Keep It Simple

Often, administrators miss the mark with workplace culture. They may expend a lot of effort every now and then or do big things in an attempt to improve morale, but they are often left without the results they were hoping for.

Why? The reason is that culture thrives in simple, consistent, everyday actions—not in grand gestures. One big annual party that lasts all night, for example, does little to repair a lack of recognition, appreciation, and genuine care exhibited during the other 364 days of the year. Big events and prizes may be nice, but they don't sustain a culture. A culture is sustained by small acts of kindness, care, and concern, and a consistency in behavior and expectations. Clarity of purpose, of standards, and of responsibilities builds an enduring workplace culture that can help you through all the challenges that will certainly come your way.

One simple thing that can dramatically shape workplace culture is knowing people's names. I know it may sound too easy, but the impact of knowing names and using them is significant. As the administrator, you must remember that you are the leader of the facility, and knowing someone's name means a lot to them! It communicates that the most important person at work (in their eyes) knows them. Get to know the names of your staff, residents, and family members as quickly as you can and continually make this a priority as new people come to your building. This simple practice will strengthen your workplace culture in big ways!

Other small things such as getting to know your staff, writing thank-you cards, or getting out from behind the desk and spending time on the floor can help you build the right culture. Think about little things you can do to show you genuinely care about the people who work for you.

One final note: don't buy into the thought that a facility's culture can't be changed quickly. It can. From day one as an administrator, there are simple things you can do to begin to change and improve the culture of your workplace. On the other hand, if you don't constantly work toward cultivating the right culture, it can change on you quickly, and you will be left wondering what happened.

Be diligent in building the right culture. Put it at the top of your priority list every day and you will be a successful administrator. Administrators in facilities without a good workplace culture typically do not last too long in the competitive skilled nursing environment.

CHAPTER 2 SUMMARY

KEY TAKEAWAYS

- Establishing the right workplace culture should be an administrator's number-one priority.
- The right culture helps attract and retain the right staff, which will lead to great clinical and financial results.
- The right workplace culture can positively impact any challenge faced at the facility.

TASKS TO EXPAND YOUR LEARNING

☐ Create a mission statement, core values, and vision statement for your facility or thoroughly review the one that already exists.

☐ Envision how you'd like your facility to run. What is it like? How do the staff act? How are the residents and family members taken care of? How do people feel as they enter your building and interact with your team? What are things the facility is accomplishing? Share this vision with your team. Ask them to go through a similar exercise and then brainstorm how to make this vision a reality.

☐ Read two leadership books that will help you establish a good culture at your facility. Some recommendations:
   1) *Be An Awesome Boss! The Four C's Model to Leadership Success* and *How Leaders can Strengthen Their Organization's Culture* by Tim Burningham
   2) *Leadership and Self-Deception* by The Arbinger Institute

3) *The Truth About Employee Engagement* and *The Five Dysfunctions of a Team* by Patrick Lencioni

☐ Interview a successful administrator and ask them about the role workplace culture plays in the success of their facility. Ask them how they go about trying to influence, impact, or change their facility's culture.

☐ Learn the names of as many staff members as you can in one week.

CHAPTER 3

Common SNF Acronyms, Abbreviations, and Terms

Introduction

If you've been around skilled nursing care much, you've heard more acronyms and abbreviations than you probably ever thought could possibly exist. These are a way of life in the health care industry, and especially in skilled nursing.

It is a good idea for administrators to familiarize themselves with the common skilled nursing–related acronyms, abbreviations, and terms listed below. Many of them you may know already. Others might be new to you, or maybe you've heard some of them before but aren't sure what they mean. Regardless, learning them will help you feel more comfortable when speaking with health care professionals and others in the industry.

Common Acronyms, Abbreviations, and Terms

AARP – American Association of Retired Persons

Ab – antibody

ABN – advance beneficiary notice

ABOM – assistant business office manager

AC – after meals

ACO – accountable care organization

ACP – advance care planning

AD – advance directive or assistive device

ADC – average daily census

ADL – activity of daily living

Ad lib – as desired

ADR – additional document request

AED – automated external defibrillator

Ag – antigen

AHCA – American Health Care Association

AI – adequate intake

AIDS – acquired immunodeficiency syndrome

AKA – above the knee amputation

AL – assisted living

ALF – assisted living facility

ALOS – average length of stay

ALS – amyotrophic lateral sclerosis

AMA – against medical advice

Amb – ambulate

AMI – acute myocardial infarction (heart attack)

a/p – anterior-posterior

APS – adult protective services

ARD – assessment reference date

AROM – active range of motion

As tol – as tolerated

AV – atrioventricular

BBP – bloodborne pathogens

BCBS – Blue Cross Blue Shield

BCLS – basic cardiac life support

BEA – below the elbow amputation

BID – two times a day

BIMS – Brief Interview for Mental Status

BIW – biweekly, twice a week

BKA – below the knee amputation

b/l – bilateral

BLS – basic life support

BM – bowel movement

BMI – body mass index

BO – business office

BOM – business office manager

BOS – base of support

BP – blood pressure

BPCI – Bundled Payments for Care Improvement

BPM – beats per minute

BSN – bachelor of science degree in nursing

BT – body temperature

BUN – blood urea nitrogen

C&S – blood culture and sensitivity

Ca – calcium

CAA – care area assessment

CABG – coronary artery bypass grafting

CAD – coronary artery disease

CAT – computerized adaptive testing

CBC – complete blood count

CBO – centralized billing office

CBS – community-based services

CCRC – continuing care retirement community

CDC – Centers for Disease Control and Prevention

CEU – continuing education unit

CF – cystic fibrosis

CFS – Cognitive Function Scale

CHD – coronary heart disease

CHF – congestive heart failure

CHO – carbohydrates

Cl – chloride

CLIA – Clinical Laboratory Improvement Amendments

CM – case manager

CMA – certified medication aide

CMP – civil monetary penalty

CMS (CMMS) – Centers for Medicare & Medicaid Services

CNA – certified nursing assistant

c/o – complaints of

CoC – change of condition

COPD – chronic obstructive pulmonary disease (cardiopulmonary disease)

COT – change of therapy

COTA – certified occupational therapy assistant

CP – care plan or cerebral palsy

CPAP – continuous positive airway pressure

CPM – continuous passive motion

CPR – cardiopulmonary resuscitation

CPS – cognitive performance score

CPT – Current Procedural Terminology

CQI – continuous quality improvement

CVA – cerebral vascular accident (stroke)

CVD – cardiovascular disease

CWF – common working file

CXR – chest x-ray

DADS – Department of Aging and Disability Services

DAT – diet as tolerated

DBP – diastolic blood pressure

d/c – discharge

DHS – Department of Human (Health) Services

DHHS – Department of Health and Human Services

DM – diabetes mellitus

DME – durable medical equipment

DNR – do not resuscitate

DOB – date of birth

DOI – date of injury

DOJ – Department of Justice

DOM – director of marketing

DON – director of nursing (nurses)

DOR – director of rehabilitation

DOS – date of surgery

DPH – Department of Public Health

DPOA – durable power of attorney

DRG – diagnosis-related group (hospital reimbursement)

DSD – director of staff development

DSO – days sales outstanding

DVT – deep vein thrombosis (blood clot)

Dx – diagnosis

E-MAR – electronic medication administration record

E-stim – electrical stimulation

E-TAR – electronic treatment administration record

EBIT – earnings before interest and taxes

EBITDAR – earnings before interest, taxes, depreciation, amortization, and rent

ECG (EKG) – electrocardiogram

ECIN – Extended Care Information Network

ED – executive director (administrator)

EDI – electronic data interchange

EEOC – Equal Employment Opportunity Commission

EMR – electronic medical record

EMS – emergency medical services

EMT – emergency medical technician

EOB – edge of bed

EOT – end of therapy

EP – elopement precautions

ETA – estimated time of arrival

Ex – exercise

Ext. – extension

FBS – fasting blood sugar

FDA – Food and Drug Administration

Fe – iron

FFS – fee for service

FI – fiscal intermediary

FMLA – Family and Medical Leave Act

FTE – full-time employee

FTT – failure to thrive

f/u – follow-up

FWB – full weight bearing

Fx – fracture

FY – fiscal year

G-tube – gastrostomy tube

GAAP – generally accepted accounting principles

GI – gastrointestinal

GNP – geriatric nurse practitioner

h – hour

H&P – history and physical

HBO – hyperbaric oxygenation

HBV – hepatitis B virus

HCA – health care association

HCPCS – Healthcare Common Procedural Coding System

HCV – hepatitis C virus

HHA – home health agency

HHS – Health and Human Services

HHSC – Health and Human Services Commission

HIC – health insurance claim

HIPAA – Health Insurance Portability and Accountability Act

HIV – human immunodeficiency virus

HMO – health maintenance (or management) organization

h/o – history of

HOB – head of bed

HR – heart rate or human resources

HS – hour of sleep

HTN – hypertension

HX – history

I&O – intake and output

I – independent

IBS – irritable bowel syndrome

ICD-10 – International Classification of Diseases, 10th Edition

ICF – intermediate care facility

ICU – intensive care unit

ID – intradermal

IDDM – insulin dependent diabetes mellitus

IDR – informal dispute resolution

IDT – interdisciplinary team

IE – initial evaluation

IJ – immediate jeopardy

IM – intramuscular

IRF – inpatient rehabilitation facility

IV – intravenous

IVP – intravenous push

J-tube – jejunostomy tube

JCAHO – Joint Commission on Accreditation of Healthcare Organizations

K – potassium

KUB – kidney, ureter, and bladder x-ray

LB – lower body

LBP – lower back pain

LE – lower extremity

LQ – lower quadrant

LMS – learning management system

LMSW – licensed medical social worker

LNHA – licensed nursing home administrator

LOC – level of care

LOS – length of stay

LPN – licensed practical nurse

Lt – left

LTAC – long-term acute care

LTC – long-term care

LTCMI – Long-Term Care Medicaid Information

LTG – long-term goal

LVN – licensed vocational nurse

MAO – Medicare Advantage organization

MAR – medication administration record

MBSS – modified barium swallow study

MCO – managed care organization

MD – doctor of medicine or muscular dystrophy

MDS – Minimum Data Set

MI – mental illness

Mod – moderate

MOM – milk of magnesia

MR – mental retardation

MRI – magnetic resonance imaging

MRSA – methicillin-resistant Staphylococcus aureus

MS – multiple sclerosis

MSDS – material safety data sheet

MSW – medical social worker

MVA – motor vehicle accident

NA – nurse aide

Na – sodium

NaCl – sodium chloride

NEO – new employee orientation

NF – nursing facility

NG tube – nasogastric tube

NH – nursing home

NHP – nursing home placement

NKA – no known allergies

NOMNC – Notice of Medicare Non-Coverage

NP – nurse practitioner

NPI – National Provider Identifier

NPO – nothing by mouth

NR – not reported

NTA – non-therapy ancillary

NWB – non-weight bearing

OASIS – Outcome and Assessment Information Set

OBRA – Omnibus Budget Reconciliation Act

OBT – over-bed table

OD – overdose

OIG – Office of Inspector General

OOB – out of bed

OPT – outpatient therapy

OR – operating room

OSHA – Occupational Safety and Health Administration

OT – occupational therapy or overtime

OTA – occupational therapy assistant

OTC – over-the-counter

OTR – occupational therapist, registered

OU – both eyes

P&L – profit and loss

P4P – pay-for-performance

PA – physician assistant

PAC – post-acute care

PASARR – Pre-Admission Screening and Annual Resident Review

PASS – pull, aim, squeeze, sweep

PBJ – payroll-based journal

PC – after meals

PCC – PointClickCare

PD – Parkinson's disease

PDF – portable document file

PDPM – Patient-Driven Payment Model

PEG tube – percutaneous endoscopic gastrostomy tube

PHI – protected health information

PIC – peripheral indwelling catheter

PICC – peripherally inserted central catheter

PIP – performance improvement plan

PLOF – prior level of function

PMH – past medical history

Pn – pain

PO – by mouth

POA – power of attorney

POC – plan of care, point of care

PLOF – prior level of function

PPD – per patient day

PPE – personal protective equipment

POS – point of service

PPO – preferred provider organization

PPS – prospective payment system

PR – by rectum

PRN – pro re nata (as needed)

PRO – peer review organization

PROM – passive range of motion

PSDA – Patient Self-Determination Act

Pt – Patient

PT – physical therapy, part-time

PTA – physical therapy assistant

PTE – part-time employee

PT INR – prothrombin time and international normalized ratio (lab test for how long it takes blood to clot)

PVC – premature ventricular contraction

PVD – peripheral vascular disease

PWB – partial weight bearing

Q – every

q2h – every 2 hours (q4h = every 4 hours, q6h = every six hours...you get the idea)

QA – quality assurance

QAPI – Quality Assurance and Performance Improvement

QI – quality improvement or quality indicators

QIC – quality improvement consultant

QID – four times per day

QIO – quality improvement organization

QIP – quality improvement plan

QM – quality of care measures

QMB – Qualified Medicare Beneficiary

QRP – quality review program

QRS – Quality Reporting System

RA – rheumatoid arthritis

RACE – rescue, alarm, contain, evacuate (or extinguish)

RAI – Resident Assessment Instrument

RAP – Resident Assessment Protocol

RBC – red blood cell

RC – related condition

RCS – Resident Classification System

RF – rehabilitation facility

RN – registered nurse

RO – regional office

r/o – rule out

ROI – return on investment

ROM – range of motion

Rot – rotation

RP – representative payee

RPh – registered pharmacist

RPT – registered physical therapist

RR – respiratory rate (breathing rate)

RRT – rapid response team

r/t – related to

Rt – right

RT – respiratory therapy or therapist

RTA – return to acute

RUG – Resource Utilization Group

RVU – relative value unit

RW – rolling walker

(S) – supervision

s/a – suicide attempt

SA – special assistance

SBA – standby assist

SI – suicidal ideation

SL – sublingual

SLP – speech language pathologist

SNF – skilled nursing facility

SNU – skilled nursing unit

SOB – shortness of breath

SOBOE – shortness of breath on exertion

SOC – standard of care

SOT – start of therapy

s/p – status post

SP – supplemental payment or suprapubic catheter

SQC – substandard quality of care

SSI – Supplemental Security Income

SSN – social security number

ST – speech therapy

STAT – at once, immediately

STG – short-term goal

SW – social worker

tag – citation or deficient practice

TAR – treatment administration record

TB – tuberculosis

TBI – traumatic brain injury

TCU – transitional care unit

THA – total hip arthroplasty

THR – total hip replacement

TIA – transient ischemic attack (mini stroke)

TID – three times per day

TIRR – The Institute for Rehabilitation and Research

Title XVIII – Medicare (Title 18 of the Social Security Act)

Title XIX – Medicaid (Title 19 of the Social Security Act)

TKA – total knee arthroplasty

TKR – total knee replacement

TO – telephone order or employee turnover

Tol – tolerated

TPN – total parenteral nutrition

TQM – total quality management

TTWB – toe-touch weight bearing

UA – urinalysis

UB – upper body

UDA – user-defined assessment

UE – upper extremity

UQ – upper quadrant

URI – upper respiratory infection

US – ultrasound

UTI – urinary tract infection

VC – verbal cues

V&S – volume and specific gravity

VA – Department of Veteran Affairs

VBP – value-based purchasing

VO – verbal order

VRE – vancomycin-resistant enterococci

WA – while awake

WB – weight bearing

WBAT – weight bearing as tolerated

WBC – white blood cell

w/c – wheelchair

WFL – within functional limits

WNL – within normal limits

y/o – years old

KEY TAKEAWAYS

- Learning common acronyms, abbreviations, and terms will build your confidence and help you understand and speak the language of the industry.

TASKS TO EXPAND YOUR LEARNING

☐ Make flashcards of the most common acronyms, abbreviations, and terms you hear but haven't quite learned. Study the flashcards until you know them well.

CHAPTER 4

Housekeeping Department

Introduction

The cleanliness of your facility sends a strong message about how you care for those within its walls. Too many administrators gloss over or ignore the issue of cleanliness and choose to focus on more "exciting" things, but don't let this be you! Understanding the basics of housekeeping goes a long way. It is well worth your time to make sure your facility is clean.

Appearance

When it comes to the physical appearance of a building, first impressions matter a lot! In fact, people will make judgments about whether your building is clean within the first minute or two of being there. For this reason, first impression areas play a key role in presenting the facility well.

First impression areas are the areas your customers and visitors see first—the parking lot and facility grounds, the lobby, the reception desk, the floors, the public restrooms, the hallways, etc. If these areas are sparkling at all times, people will assume the same for the rest of the building. However, if your first impression areas are dirty, dusty, unkempt, and cluttered, people will assume the entire facility is the same way—even if the patient rooms are immaculate.

To make sure first impression areas always look great, housekeepers must routinely "police" them. Policing is when a housekeeper swings by and spot cleans an area, such as emptying the trash and cleaning a toilet seat in a public restroom or organizing the magazines and straightening up the furniture in the lobby. Remember, policing does not require thorough cleaning. Whereas most rooms in a facility are cleaned once a day, your first impression areas should be policed multiple times throughout the day and spot cleaned as needed.

Another way to improve the appearance of first impression areas is by strongly encouraging every employee in the facility to never walk by a piece of trash on the floor without stopping to pick it up. Imagine how clean the facility would appear if all employees never left a piece of trash or a spill they encounter on the floor without taking care of it. This should be the goal. As the administrator, you should make this expectation very clear. You should also lead by example by never, ever walking by a spill or piece of trash on the floor without taking care of it.

One other tip is that the floors are the most important part of any area. People tend to look down and notice floors before anything else. If the floors look clean and shiny, most people will trust that the entire facility (not just the floors) is clean and shiny. That's why having a strong and consistent floor maintenance program—including stripping, waxing, and buffing hard floors or cleaning, removing stains, and extracting carpet floors—is so important. For example, all floors should be buffed or vacuumed regularly: high-traffic areas more frequently, and low-traffic areas less frequently. Floors go a long way in setting the tone for your building in terms of the overall appearance and perception of cleanliness.

Infection Control

Though maintaining first impression areas is critical, this doesn't mean that other areas can be ignored and not cleaned. In fact, just the opposite is true. Preventing the spread of infection is the duty of all health care institutions, and good housekeeping practices are vital in this regard. It is very important to have a team that is trained to be attentive and clean even the most minor areas of a patient room. For example, "high touch" areas, which include TV remotes, door handles, phones, sink faucets, call buttons, bedrails, and furniture handles, are often overlooked but are the most important to clean in order to ensure proper infection control. These are areas that are most often touched by multiple people throughout the day and therefore must be sanitized regularly.

Overflowing trash cans on nursing carts and in resident rooms are also a common occurrence and can increase the likelihood of spreading infections. Training team members to quickly remove trash when full will not only prevent a common eyesore found in many SNFs, but will also help with controlling the spread of disease.

Failing to have good cleanliness and infection control practices can lead to huge consequences in a SNF. Remember, you are housing a vulnerable population whose health is often already compromised. Therefore, well-trained and diligent housekeeping team members are a must.

Finally, while we are on the topic, the number one way to prevent the spread of infection is by thorough hand washing. Ensuring staff wash and sanitize their hands frequently is a must! Pay attention while you're walking the halls of your facility and make sure staff are regularly and properly washing their hands.

KEY TAKEAWAYS

- First impression areas set the tone and create the customer's perception of the cleanliness of the entire facility.
- Floors are typically the first thing people notice when they walk into a room, and their condition forms the perception of the facility's overall cleanliness.
- High-touch areas in rooms, such as light switches and TV remotes, must be cleaned often.
- Good cleaning prevents infections from spreading and will keep staff and patients safe.
- Proper handwashing is the number one way to avoid the spread of infection.
- Implementing simple systems to inspect and maintain the cleanliness of your building can help ensure a very clean building.

TASKS TO EXPAND YOUR LEARNING

- ☐ Walk into a store, restaurant, physician's office, or other business and decide within a minute or two if you believe it is clean or not. What made you feel one way or another? What can you learn from this exercise to improve the perception of cleanliness in your facility?
- ☐ Inspect the cleanliness of a patient room after it has just been cleaned. Look at high-touch areas in the room to make sure they have been sanitized.
- ☐ Check your busiest first impression areas, such as the public restroom or front lobby, every two hours

throughout the day. What do you notice? Are you always starting with a great first impression?

☐ Walk the halls of your building and count the number of staff you notice washing their hands.

COMMON POSITIONS IN THE DEPARTMENT

Housekeeping director or supervisor – Leads the housekeeping team and is responsible for ordering housekeeping supplies, managing staff, overseeing the budget, preparing schedules, and maintaining the overall cleanliness and appearance of the facility. This person is typically a working supervisor, meaning they don't just sit in an office and do paperwork, but they have assigned cleaning areas and are on the floor mopping, wiping walls, dusting, etc.

Housekeeping aide – Normally given a designated area to clean each day. Takes out trash, cleans rooms and common areas, sweeps, mops, dusts, sanitizes, etc.

Floor tech – Follows a routine to buff floors and do daily maintenance on them. Strips and waxes floors as needed.

CHAPTER 5

Laundry Department

Introduction

Clean linen that looks and smells great is the key deliverable of a successful laundry department. Torn sheets, stained linen, and missing clothing are probably the most common complaints faced by laundry departments. Having team members who are organized, hardworking, and able to follow clear systems is important to maintaining a well-run laundry program.

Two Secrets to Success

When it comes to laundry services, there are two factors that will win the day: appearance and smell.

Imagine you're being admitted to a hospital. Just before you get plopped down on a bed, you notice some serious stains on the sheets. Though you aren't sure, they appear to be stains from either blood or feces. How comfortable will you be sleeping in that bed tonight, and how you will you feel about the hospital?

Now imagine instead that to your delight, the sheets appear sparkling clean. As you settle in, however, you notice a funky smell. Maybe it's mold, or maybe it's something worse—you aren't sure. You bring the bed sheet up to your face to mask the smell and then you realize: it's the sheets that smell! Again, how comfortable will you be sleeping in that bed, and how will you feel about the hospital you just were admitted to?

As you can imagine, your customers can be quickly turned off by stained or less-than-fresh-smelling linen. In fact, this can sour their entire stay. However, if you can consistently provide linen that both looks and smells good, most of your customers will be satisfied with your laundry services. An administrator should pay close attention to those two factors.

Personal Laundry

Most facilities provide free laundry services for residents and patients, however they also allow family members to take their loved ones' clothes home and do the laundry themselves. The same is true for linen. Some families and/or patients prefer to use their own linen from home, but most will opt to use the linen provided by the facility.

Effective systems and processes are needed to make sure that resident clothing is laundered professionally and returned in a timely manner. One very important system in the laundry department is how resident clothing is labeled. Being able to identify what belongs to who is probably the biggest battle most laundry departments face. Ensuring articles of clothing are all labeled appropriately before they go to the laundry room is crucial, and can save a lot of headaches.

Other Things to Consider

There are many important cross-contamination and infection control measures a facility must take when handling laundry. For example, dirty linen must never be mixed with or even be in the same room as the clean linen while being laundered. Also, the laundry room must be kept clean and tidy and free from dust and debris. Finally, an important safety item to watch for is excessive lint in the dryers' lint traps. Lint is very combustible, so lint traps must be cleaned frequently.

When state surveyors come to your building for the annual health inspection survey, they will inspect the laundry room. They will look specifically at overall cleanliness, organization, infection control measures, and they will always check for excessive lint.

KEY TAKEAWAYS

- The appearance and smell of linen create the strongest perception of a facility's laundry services.
- An effective system for labeling clothes will save you from numerous complaints and headaches.
- Keeping clean and dirty linen separate at all times prevents the spread of infection. This practice will be monitored closely by regulatory visitors.
- During the annual health inspection survey, surveyors will always check the laundry room. It must be kept clean, tidy, and free of debris and excessive lint.

TASKS TO EXPAND YOUR LEARNING

- ☐ Inspect your laundry room and rate it based on cleanliness and organization.
- ☐ Pick three patient rooms and inspect the linen in those rooms. Does it appear clean and fresh?
- ☐ Go to a clean linen closet and smell the linen. What perception does the scent of your linen provide?
- ☐ Look at the clean resident clothing in the laundry room and see if the clothing is clearly labeled with the name of the person it belongs to.

COMMON POSITIONS IN THE DEPARTMENT

Housekeeping and laundry director or supervisor – In nearly every facility, the laundry department is led by either the housekeeping supervisor or the maintenance director. They assume responsibility for the department, with duties such as ordering supplies and linen, managing staff, overseeing the department's budget, preparing schedules, ensuring proper infection control protocols, and maintaining the overall quality of the laundry services.

Laundry aide – Washes dirty laundry. Folds clean laundry. Transports clothing to and from the laundry room. Delivers resident clothing to rooms and stocks clean linen in the linen closets. Maintains the cleanliness of the laundry area and communicates supply needs to the supervisor. Laundry aides may also have some housekeeping assignments.

CHAPTER 6

Maintenance Department

Introduction

The physical upkeep of a facility can be a big task, and it is usually handled by one or two team members. In order to be successful, these individuals must be organized and able to effectively prioritize the often long list of items that need to be taken care of.

Likewise, all of a facility's team members need to understand their responsibility in identifying and reporting maintenance needs. Too frequently, small problems with simple fixes go ignored. This can really turn off customers and visitors. For example, an unchanged light bulb or a detached towel rack in a patient restroom can create a negative perception. However, if staff is diligent in reporting such issues and the maintenance team handles them in a timely manner, the building will maintain a good appearance.

In addition to a high level of communication between team members and departments, consistent use of plant maintenance systems such as project logs and maintenance logs can help ensure the upkeep and appearance of the building.

First Impressions

As we learned in Chapter 4, first impression areas are very important to the overall perception of the upkeep of your facility. If your first impression areas need painting, have chipped floor tiles, or are missing outlet covers, for example, visitors will assume that the facility is poorly maintained—even if that isn't the reality. Therefore, maintenance needs in first impression areas may require higher prioritization than those in lesser-seen areas such as linen closets, utility rooms, or even offices, although the upkeep of the entire facility is important.

Additionally, when considering how to spend capital expenditure dollars and doing facility remodels and upgrades, you will get more bang for your buck—or a greater return on investment—by starting with first impression areas. The reality is that most potential customers won't have any interest in how nice the resident restroom is if the front lobby is unappealing and outdated.

Maintenance Contractors

From A/C and washer/dryer repairs to hiring refrigerator and freezer techs, plumbers, electricians, roofers, and more, the costs of maintenance contractors can add up quickly and substantially. For this reason, it is important to realize that not all maintenance directors and maintenance techs are created equally. Those with higher skill sets, who can handle more repairs instead of having to call in vendors, can be of great benefit to your facility.

Frequently evaluating the maintenance team's skills and improving and expanding them can be a good investment. And sometimes hiring and paying more for maintenance personnel with extra skills ends up being more cost-effective than calling in vendors all the time for repairs. Since the maintenance and repair needs among different facilities vary greatly, there is no one-size-fits-all strategy for how to best address these needs. But, as an administrator, evaluating the skills needed of your maintenance staff from time to time is a good practice.

Preventative Maintenance

Preventative maintenance—proactively maintaining and fixing things before they become a problem— is also a great way to save time and money. Though this practice requires an upfront investment, the returns are far greater. For example, changing the batteries in smoke detectors on a routine basis rather than as needed can save time and ensure the detectors are always in good working order. The facilities with the best results in plant maintenance are those that invest in great preventative maintenance systems and programs.

With today's technology, there are plenty of electronic programs and software out there to help with preventative maintenance and the overall upkeep of your facility. When utilized properly, these programs often are worth the investment.

Other Important Tasks

On top of being responsible for the general maintenance and upkeep of the facility, there are two other significant tasks often assigned to the maintenance department:

1. **Adhering to the life safety code.** In addition to an annual health survey, your facility will also undergo an annual survey to ensure compliance with all the rules and regulations in the life safety code. And just so you know, the life safety code book is extremely thick! While studying up on these rules and regulations is a good idea, hiring a maintenance director who has experience with and knowledge of these rules and regulations is even better.
2. **Overseeing the emergency preparedness and disaster plan.** In response to numerous major natural disasters in the United States in recent years, SNFs now face heightened scrutiny about emergency preparedness planning, plus more rules and regulations. It is vital to have robust and comprehensive plans in place so your facility will be ready in the event of an emergency. This plan should be reviewed often, and training must be given to the staff on how to access the plan and properly respond in the event of an emergency. Typically, a copy of the plan is kept at each nurses

station, the administrators office, and the maintenance office at a minimum.

When it comes to making sure your plans are sufficient, local emergency preparedness experts and even other facilities can offer valuable help and guidance. A good plan is a must for all facilities!

Conclusion

As you can see, the maintenance department plays an important role in the success and safety of your building. As the administrator, it is important you review and ensure proper maintenance systems and plans are always in place.

KEY TAKEAWAYS

- Everyone needs to pitch in to identify and communicate the building's maintenance needs.
- The upkeep and appearance of first impression areas shape the perception of the upkeep of the entire facility.
- Preventative maintenance programs are important and will save you time and money.
- In addition to the upkeep of the facility, the maintenance department often has other important responsibilities, such as adhering to life safety rules and regulations and overseeing the emergency preparedness and disaster plan.

TASKS TO EXPAND YOUR LEARNING

- ☐ Visit a store, restaurant, physician's office or other business and determine if the building is well-maintained. Evaluate how you came to your conclusion and what it might mean for your facility.
- ☐ Ask staff members how they report items that need to be repaired. Also ask them how they know when a problem they've reported has been fixed.
- ☐ Make a list of vendors commonly used by the maintenance department and analyze how much the facility has spent on each over the past year. Based on this information, what skills might be valuable for your maintenance staff to have?

☐ Review the emergency preparedness and disaster plan carefully on your own. Is there anything that is unclear, confusing, or missing? Ensure that everyone knows how to access the disaster plan manual in the event of an emergency.

COMMON POSITIONS IN THE DEPARTMENT

Maintenance director or supervisor – Oversees and ensures the upkeep of the building. He or she is responsible for compliance with life safety codes and regulations, and most often maintains and updates the facility's emergency preparedness and disaster plan. He or she is responsible for the department's budget, ordering supplies, doing or facilitating repairs, and managing any maintenance contractors or vendors used by the facility (such as an A/C repairman, for example). This person is normally a working supervisor who completes projects and does front-line work such as changing a doorknob, painting a room, replacing a light bulb, etc. He or she is also usually responsible for the maintenance and repairs of medical equipment and furniture. In many facilities, the maintenance director will oversee the housekeeping and laundry staff. It's common for a maintenance director to be a one-person department, while others may have techs or assistants.

Maintenance tech – Acts as a helper to the maintenance director and completes tasks as assigned.

Assistant maintenance director or supervisor – Though rare, this position is for an individual who would otherwise be a maintenance tech but has the necessary leadership abilities and skill set to handle some paperwork, matters related to life safety regulations, and other higher-level tasks, in addition to manual labor. This individual completes tasks as assigned by the maintenance director.

Floor tech – Routinely buffs floors and does daily maintenance and upkeep on them. Strips and waxes floors as needed. (This position often falls under the housekeeping department, but it can also be assigned to the maintenance department).

CHAPTER 7

Dietary Services

Introduction

For many of your residents, mealtime is the most enjoyable part of the day. In fact, the quality of the dining experience will often mirror residents' perceived quality of life at the facility. Thus, dietary services are not only important for health and nutrition but also for the overall contentment and well-being of your residents.

Presentation, Temperature, and Smell

Some vital things to consider for your meal service are presentation, temperature, and smell. Though you'd think taste would be at the top of the list of things that make a meal enjoyable, there are other factors that sometimes play a bigger role (especially for the elderly, who often slowly lose their ability to taste).

The way a meal is presented on a plate is critically important. If the food looks appetizing, regardless of its taste, it will often get praised. A meal that looks unappetizing, even if it is delicious, will often go untouched or be deemed unsatisfactory. Enhancing the presentation of your food will go a long way in pleasing your guests.

The temperature of the food also plays a big role in how much residents enjoy it. Cold eggs, for example, just aren't the same as warm ones. Having systems in place to make sure residents are served food at an appropriate temperature is vital. Food temperature is perhaps the number-one complaint received by most dietary departments in a SNF.

Finally, the smell of the food is crucial. We all know smells have a way of impacting the taste of our food. If things smell good, we eat and often enjoy them. When they don't, it is a totally different story. Serving foods that have pleasant aromas and avoiding others that don't smell so nice is a good idea. Likewise, being cognizant of smells other than food in your facility, particularly where residents eat, is important.

Unfortunately, food presentation, temperature, and smell are often overlooked or ignored in SNFs, even though controlling these factors goes a long way in influencing residents' perception of the food and overall dining experience. So, if you find yourself struggling to please your customers with your meal services, or are receiving a lot of complaints during mealtimes, taking a close look at these three considerations is a great place to start.

Enhancing the Dining Experience

Besides the food itself, there are many other factors that can enhance the dining experience at your facility. How is the meal offered and presented to the residents? What food choices and options are given? What do residents do as they wait for food to be served? What is the atmosphere of your dining areas like? All of these are things to consider in creating a great dining experience.

There's no lack of alternative ways to enhance the dining experience. From restaurant-style to fine dining to made-to-order services, or even to family-style (meals are served in large dishes; residents pass the food around the table and serve themselves just like at home), there are many approaches to serving meals in a delightful and pleasing way. Get creative and ask your customers often how they are feeling about the dining experience.

Facilities that offer great dining services are able to separate themselves from their competitors and can advertise this distinction as a reason for customers to choose their facility over others. Though this may seem a little far-fetched, you'd be surprised by how far promises of good food and meal services can go with many potential customers. Develop a reputation for providing great meals and your census will likely increase.

Snacks

Snacks are also an important part of residents' nutrition and quality of life. And snacks are something regulators love to look closely at so don't forget to make sure they are appetizing and available. Too often snacks are never handed out or they are stored in a way that makes them unappealing to eat. Monitoring appropriate temperatures of snacks is another item that is often overlooked.

Diets

In the skilled nursing setting, different dietary requirements abound. Between no added salt, pureed foods, allergies, and so on, keeping diets straight can be a challenge. But it is crucial! In some instances, not adhering to residents' dietary needs appropriately can cause major problems—including death, in the most extreme example. As an administrator, you must make certain your facility always has a strong and consistent system of communication in place between nursing and dietary services.

Serving Meals

Now, with all the food talk out of the way, what is important to know about the actual inner workings of the dietary department? Serving food to a large group of people certainly has its challenges. Finding efficient ways to prepare and serve meals is necessary. But every kitchen is different, and every facility has different equipment, layouts, floor plans, etc. so unfortunately there is no magic formula or surefire way to best prepare and serve meals. That said, gathering and listening to your guests' feedback about their dining experience and frequently analyzing your facility's methods and systems for food delivery is important for your dietary department's success.

Controlling Costs

As you might guess, food expenses are among a SNF's highest costs. There is a lot you can do to minimize food costs such as look at and compare different vendors' prices, prepare more meals from scratch, and pick up essentials at the local grocery store as some examples. However, in my experience, the number-one way to control food costs is to minimize food waste. So much food is never eaten, never touched, and simply gets thrown out. When this happens, it is like throwing money into a trash can.

The good news is that there are strategies for minimizing food waste. The first is understanding your residents' food preferences or likes and dislikes. If Mr. Jones hates milk, for example, why is he being served milk three times a day? Or if Ms. Smith doesn't eat pork, why does bacon and sausage end up on her plate each morning?

Your dietary supervisor should meet with each new resident within 24 hours of their arrival. The purpose of this meeting is to learn the resident's likes and dislikes so he or she can be served accordingly. These preferences should be updated quarterly at a minimum, because they do change. The dietary supervisor should also constantly monitor food waste and approach residents who seem to not be eating certain items to learn if their preferences have changed.

The second strategy for reducing food waste is paying attention to portion sizes. Many dietary departments serve food somewhat haphazardly: one resident will receive a giant spoonful of mashed potatoes, while another resident only gets two bites' worth. Make sure serving utensils are appropriately matched with the food that is being served, and that staff is trained on how to dish out correct portion sizes. This will cut down on waste.

These two strategies, more than any others, will save you money by effectively reducing waste.

Regulatory Considerations

From a regulatory standpoint, the kitchen is always a hot spot. Nearly every time a surveyor enters your building, he or she will check the kitchen, and during the annual survey process the kitchen and meal services will be scrutinized closely.

Cleanliness and sanitation in the kitchen is a commonly cited and deficient practice. Buildup on pots and pans, dust in high places, rust on a can opener, grease in corners or on surface edges, and debris hiding under appliances are all common findings. Your kitchen must be kept as spotless as possible not just for regulatory reasons, but most importantly for the health and well-being of those you serve.

Survey teams also closely review and monitor for appropriate temperatures for both hot and cold food serving and storage, proper labeling and dating of food, the presence of expired food, and dishwashing temperatures and procedures.

The bottom line: it's important as an administrator to visit your kitchen often to make sure its conditions are always in good order.

KEY TAKEAWAYS

- Meals are often the most important part of a resident's day, and thus must be exceptional.
- Food presentation, temperature, and smell are three major often-forgotten factors that play a significant role in customer satisfaction with dining services.
- When it comes to residents' dietary needs, a strong system of communication between departments is crucial. This system must be reviewed often for effectiveness and thoroughness. Serving the wrong diet to a resident even once can result in a negative and possibly dangerous outcome.
- Controlling food waste is often the best way to control food costs.
- Dietary services are heavily scrutinized during annual surveys and other regulatory visits, and are very commonly cited for deficiencies.

TASKS TO EXPAND YOUR LEARNING

- ☐ Eat a breakfast, lunch, and dinner meal in your facility's dining room and rate the dining experience.
- ☐ Enter the dining room during a meal and rate the presentation of the food. Also rate the fragrance in the room.
- ☐ Observe the preparation of plates. Are portion sizes consistent?
- ☐ Observe the dishwashing process. How much food is thrown away?

COMMON POSITIONS IN THE DEPARTMENT

Dietary supervisor – Oversees the meal service and dining experience and ensures that dietary needs are met for all residents. Manages the kitchen and ensures proper sanitation. Oversees the ordering, stocking, and storage of food, and that all regulations are followed. Ensures the quality of the food being served and works within specified budgets. In most states, the dietary supervisor must have a certification.

Cook – Primarily prepares and cooks meals but may take on other assignments in the kitchen as needed.

Dietary aide – Assists cook with meal preparation, prepares trays, cleans kitchen, and does other tasks as needed to ensure high-quality service.

Dishwasher – Cleans, sanitizes, and washes dishes after meal services. Helps in the kitchen as needed.

Dietician consultant – Observes, reviews, and monitors diets to ensure that proper nutritional needs are met. Ensures dietary regulations pertaining to resident dietary reviews are met. Makes recommendations to changes of resident diets and diet related physician orders as appropriate. Helps recommend and create menus for proper nutrition. Inspects kitchen sanitation.

Typically, a facility's dietary supervisor is not a dietician, thus requiring the need for a consultant. A dietician consultant is not at the facility every day, but more commonly is there once a week or maybe two or three times a month depending on the number of residents and the needs of the facility. The dietician consultant is normally not employed by the facility and works under a contract.

CHAPTER 8

Activities Department

Introduction

Just as with mealtimes, activities can be events residents really look forward to. Creating memorable experiences with activities should be your goal.

Activity programs vary widely among facilities. Some are great and provide a lot of fun, satisfaction, and happiness in residents' lives, and others are lackluster at best. Ensuring you have a good activity program will bless the lives of those you serve.

Activity Program

What constitutes a good activity program? Ask your residents! Sometimes facilities don't give residents enough say about what kinds of activities they'd enjoy. Getting their feedback is really the best way to design a successful activity program. People like different things—you might be surprised by what your residents would like to do.

That being said, sometimes residents don't know what types of activities they might like or enjoy. You should be creative and find different ways to engage your customers. Activities such as playing video games or providing a service to others might not seem too appealing to your residents at first, but often end up being the best of all. Your activities director should get to know the residents and find out what their interests and likes are, and then cater a program to them.

Holidays are a great excuse to have parties and celebrate. Make sure your activity program includes holiday celebrations for your residents. Whether it's Halloween, Mother's Day, or Christmas, holiday activities have a way of bringing people together and encouraging them to have fun. Holiday activities can be some of the most memorable for those at your facility.

Enriching Your Program

Strong activity programs often include a volunteer network. Volunteers can do so much to enhance and expand your activities. Whether they're establishing a book club, doing arts and crafts, teaching a skill, or putting together performance groups, there are often many individuals in the community who love to share their interests and talents and are willing to volunteer their time. Your activities director should regularly work on cultivating a strong base of volunteers.

Facility outings can also be enjoyable. These can include, for instance, going out to lunch at a nearby restaurant, enjoying a movie or show, taking a shopping trip to Walmart, or going fishing at a local pond. Find opportunities to take your residents on outings—they usually like to get out and have fun.

Normally, people's desire to give back and help others doesn't go away. Though often our residents are dependent on others for their care, they can still serve and help others as well. I've found that service-related activities are some of the activities residents enjoy most. Putting together hygiene kits for victims of a natural disaster, crocheting and knitting blankets for a local pediatric ICU, and writing notes of appreciation to staff members are examples of activities that enable residents to serve others. These types of projects will enrich your activity program.

Entertainment

One of the biggest expenses in an activities department budget can be the cost of entertainers. Some facilities pay large sums of money each month to hire musicians and other entertainers to perform. It's a great thing to do—entertainers can really liven up your activity program and should not be overlooked.

What if your budget doesn't allow for much live entertainment? Should you just forget about it? No! Often, local churches, schools, and other community clubs have performance groups that are very good at what they do and will jump at the chance to perform at your facility.

Likewise, many professional entertainers may volunteer or be willing to perform at your facility for only a small fee. It certainly never hurts to ask. Your activities director should actively seek out quality entertainment that the facility can afford.

Added Value

A good activity program can take strain and stress off both residents and caregivers. When activities are well-attended and enjoyed by many, caregivers get a break from providing labor-intensive care: it's a relief for them to participate in an enjoyable activity with the residents instead of doing their usual running from room to room to answer call lights and attend to needs.

Activities can also divert a resident's attention away from their normal worries, stresses, and anxieties and give them a chance to relax and enjoy life. Overall, the activity program can add significant value to a facility.

Regulatory Considerations

There are a few important things to consider when looking at the regulations around activities.

First, activities should be varied to meet the interests of a diverse patient population. Surveyors will not look too kindly upon programs that exclusively have Bingo scheduled all day, every day for example.

Second, activity listings should be posted, and residents should be made aware of them including when they will take place. Often, facilities put a large monthly activities calendar in a highly-visible place for all to see. It is also common to have monthly activities calendars in each resident room.

Finally, activities should also be provided on the weekends, and "after hours" activities should take place from time to time.

Resident Council

Typically, the activities director organizes and supports the resident council. The resident council is a group of residents that meets regularly (usually monthly) to discuss any needs, concerns, or issues in the facility. Any resident should be allowed to attend the meetings.

The resident council usually has officers such as a president, vice president, and secretary; these officers help lead the council discussions and meetings. The activities director takes notes and documents discussions during these meetings. He or she shares concerns and meeting minutes with the administrator, director of nursing, and other key department heads as needed.

Resident council meetings are important, and the administrator should ask if he or she can attend from time to time. (Note that facility staff members, including the administrator, must be invited in order to attend. This is the residents' meeting after all, and no one is allowed to show up uninvited.)

During annual surveys, the surveyors will attend a resident council meeting and ask questions about many different aspects of the facility, such as care, staff, safety, and food. Comments from this resident council will often be cited when deficiencies or citations are written.

Assessments

Your activities director must do an activities assessment with each new resident who enters the building. The activities director should also update the assessment quarterly at a minimum to ensure the activities program is meeting each residents' needs.

Residents who are bedbound or not interested in large group activities should still be offered activities they can do on their own—and these should be more than just watching TV or listening to music. There are plenty of activities for bedbound individuals that can improve their quality of life as well as their health and well-being. These in-room activities are also looked at closely by surveyors during the annual survey process.

Though activities are a smaller part of an administrator's focus in comparison to other areas, they are still vital to the facility. Ensuring that you have a solid activity program will go a long way toward your facility's success.

KEY TAKEAWAYS

- Creating memorable experiences should be the goal of every activity.
- A strong volunteer network can greatly enhance your activity program.
- A good activity program helps in more ways than you might think, including taking strain off caregivers and clinical team members.
- Activity programs must include weekend activities, cater to different interests, and offer in-room activities for those who don't attend activities outside of their room.

TASKS TO EXPAND YOUR LEARNING

- ☐ Look at your facility's activities calendar and identify the most frequent activity provided for residents. Ask several residents if they enjoy that activity.
- ☐ Go to an activity and determine if it is well-attended. Also observe how staff interact with the residents during the activity. Brainstorm ideas for making activities better-attended.
- ☐ Google *bedbound activities* and create a list of 25 different activities that can be done with bedbound residents.

COMMON POSITIONS IN THE DEPARTMENT

Activities director – Oversees the activities department. Establishes and coordinates the activity program and most resident parties and events. Conducts activities assessments and ensures that the facility is meeting all rules and regulations pertaining to activities. Manages the activities budget. Participates in in-room activities with residents who may be bedbound or unwilling to leave their room. Leads the facility's volunteer program. Helps organize, coordinate, and takes notes at resident council meetings. Supervises other activity personnel. The activities director must be certified per your state's rules and regulations.

Activities aide or assistant – Helps the activities director complete their assignments and often leads, coordinates, and oversees different activities throughout the day. Participates in in-room activities as assigned.

CHAPTER 9

Social Services

Introduction

The duties and responsibilities of social services can vary greatly among facilities based on the needs of residents, families, and the community. The social services tasks in a SNF are normally handled by one individual who is a licensed social worker. There are certain circumstances or special situations per state and federal regulations that would allow a facility to have a social services director or social services representative that is not licensed, however most SNFs must employ a licensed social worker per regulations.

A good social worker can save the administrator and other team members a lot of headaches. The most effective SNF social workers are great communicators and are very organized. They also are individuals who are skilled at handling difficult problems and situations.

Seven Common Social Services Roles

Though the role of a social worker depends on the facility's unique needs, there are some universal—and very important— responsibilities social workers typically undertake.

1. **Discharge planning.** A social worker helps with the process of discharging patients to their homes or to other settings, such as an assisted living facility. A high level of organization and communication is needed for discharges to go smoothly.

   There are typically a lot of moving parts during the discharge process, and many people are involved and need to stay informed, such as the resident, physician, nurse, family members, and the pharmacy staff—just to mention a few. Overseeing the process and ensuring the successful execution of each discharge is an important responsibility for most social workers in skilled nursing. Keep in mind that the discharge process is the last impression the facility will leave with a customer who is returning to the community. It isn't uncommon for a poor discharge to sour an otherwise great experience at a facility.

2. **Care plan meetings.** Care plan meetings are an important process in a SNF. A care plan meeting is a chance to create an individualized plan of care that includes input from the individual, physician, family, and caregivers. A good care plan meeting keeps everyone informed and helps the patient receive the best care possible.

   These meetings are held frequently with each resident and their families (normally upon admission and then quarterly thereafter at a minimum). They are typically led by the social services director and also include other members of the leadership team.

   The social services director sets the tone for these important meetings. They ensure all concerns, team member involvement, and communication before, after and during the meeting are handled in a professional and supportive manner. In many instances, care plan meetings play an extremely important role to the customer's overall experience with your facility.

3. **Overseeing the facility's grievance and theft and loss logs and systems.** A grievance log is a log of complaints or concerns that any resident or family member expresses to the facility. It includes the date of the grievance as well as the resolution of the grievance. The theft and loss log is a log of any items reported as stolen or lost. This log also includes the date the missing item was reported and the resolution. The grievance and theft and loss systems are the processes and steps the facility takes to investigate, report, and resolve any grievances or theft and loss.

    Both systems and both logs are very important in a SNF for a few reasons. One reason is nearly every time a surveyor walks into your building, including during the annual survey process, they will want to see a copy of the grievance log to ensure the facility is recording, investigating, and resolving concerns in a timely and appropriate manner. Another reason is when these systems and logs are managed well, customer satisfaction improves.

    To manage these systems well, grievances as well as theft and loss situations should be addressed and resolved quickly and effectively. A critical piece of this is good communication and follow-up with all involved. It is also important for the social services director to be very responsive and proactive. A recurring problem on the grievance log such as multiple residents complaining about cold food over an extended period can lead to bigger issues.

    It is important to remember that when these logs and systems are not handled well, it opens the door for a lot of problems, including dissatisfied customers and regulatory scrutiny, tags, and fines.

4. **Maintaining and verifying code status for each resident.** Upon admission, the facility must establish a code status, which is whether the resident would like to be resuscitated or not in the event they stop breathing. A DNR (do not resuscitate) or full code (do resuscitate) instructs staff how to handle such situations. Resuscitation in the elderly population can be very traumatic and often causes serious health complications. A social worker or other facility member should thoroughly explain the risks and benefits of both options and then ensure the resident's wishes are made clear.

5. **Helping to safeguard resident rights.** A solid understanding of the rights of residents, plus understanding the issue of abuse and its prevention, is important. Often the social worker will provide regular training, information, and reminders to facility staff about these very important topics.

6. **Document, document, document.** Just about any conversation a social worker has with a resident or family member can and should be documented. A social worker's documentation can really help paint a clear picture of the needs of the resident as well as how the facility is working to address and meet those needs. Poor documentation from a social worker can put a facility at great risk. The administrator and director of nursing should review social services notes from time to time and, as necessary, offer the social worker feedback and training on proper documentation.

7. **Work closely with the facility-assigned ombudsperson.**
The social services director often has the closest and
most well-established relationship with the facility
ombudsperson. Working to develop a strong working
relationship of trust and confidence with this appointed
resident advocate is another typical and important role.
(More information about the ombudsperson can be
found in Chapter 17.)

Final Thoughts

A social worker's other common responsibilities may involve
doing regular resident assessments and interviews (including
conducting interviews and investigations about certain
allegations or problems that arise), helping residents apply for
Medicaid benefits, scheduling and coordinating certain services
such as psychological or dental care, explaining insurance
benefits and community programs or community assistance
that may aid residents or their families, and helping to conduct
customer satisfaction surveys.

Social workers can burn out easily because they often carry
the weight of everyone's problems on their shoulders, so be
sure to keep a close eye on them. Share your appreciation for
them often, point out all the good they do for the facility and
for others, and make sure they get uninterrupted breaks
throughout their day. A good social worker is a huge asset to a
SNF.

KEY TAKEAWAYS

- Social services can have a wide range of duties and responsibilities and can add a lot of value to the facility.
- Social workers need to be great communicators and work well with a diverse group of individuals.
- Key responsibilities of social services include discharge planning, overseeing care plan meetings, maintaining the grievance and theft and loss systems and logs, and confirming code status.
- Thorough documentation from a social worker is extremely important.

TASKS TO EXPAND YOUR LEARNING

☐ Participate in a care plan meeting. How did your team interact with the family? Were concerns resolved, questions answered, and care plans made clear? Was the care plan meeting a positive experience for everyone involved?

☐ Handle a grievance and a theft and loss concern on your own. Do an investigation and work with others to resolve the problem.

☐ List the top three most common grievances and the top three most common items reported lost at the facility over the last six months. Develop a plan to minimize these top complaints and losses.

☐ Build a stronger relationship by calling your facility's ombudsperson and asking them about their role and responsibilities. Also ask them what they believe is

important for administrators to know and do as the
leader of the facility.

☐ Review the facility's resident rights and provide a
training to your staff about them.

COMMON POSITIONS IN THE DEPARTMENT

Social services director or social worker – Coordinates
discharges, leads care plan meetings, and is often responsible
for tracking, documenting, and resolving grievances and theft
and loss issues. Ensures that the needs of the residents are
being met and that their rights are being honored. Performs
interviews, assessments, and investigations. Documents often,
and has a high level of communication with families, colleagues,
and others. Typically holds many other responsibilities as
designated by the needs of the facility and the residents and
their families.

Social services assistant – Helps the social services director with
their duties and fulfills responsibilities as assigned. Many
facilities do not have an assistant.

CHAPTER 10

Medical Records

Introduction

Meticulous documentation and recordkeeping has become as vital a part of the skilled nursing industry as any. Good organization—and the leadership of a highly organized medical records director—is crucial to the success of a medical records department in a SNF.

Roles

The medical records department plays a key role in ensuring documentation is thorough and complete. In order to participate in Medicare, Medicaid, and other programs, there are many documents that must be processed in a thorough and timely manner with all the necessary dates and signatures.

A good medical records director will help the facility stay on top of, and in compliance with, all of the necessary forms and rules pertaining to medical records. They recognize that not dotting every "i" or crossing every "t" can result in non-payment or takebacks of payment from the facility. For this reason, reviewing clinical records during daily prospective payment system (PPS) meetings and other meetings is important (more to come on these meetings in Chapter 25).

In our highly digitized world, medical records personnel often spend time scanning important documents into the EMR (electronic medical record). Though this task can be mundane, it is vital to ensuring that records are up-to-date, accurate, and complete. If a record is missing the latest information and documentation, it can lead to poor quality care.

At any given moment, a medical record may be requested for review. Therefore, it is important for the medical records director to make sure the facility's records are always current and able to be quickly retrieved. Common reasons why medical records might be requested include visits from surveyors or representatives from other government agencies, additional document requests (ADRs) by different payers, or lawyers seeking possible litigation, to name a few.

The medical records department plays a key role in communication among departments. For example, when new physician orders are written pertaining to multiple departments, the medical records department will help ensure that everyone is made aware of them.

Census information and accuracy may also be overseen by the medical records department. This is important not only for care, but also for billing purposes.

Auditing charts to verify appropriate documentation and closing charts after the patient has discharged are other important functions of the medical records department. Additionally, this department tracks down physicians for signatures, and is responsible for confidentiality and the safekeeping of records.

Complete Records

Reviewers, surveyors, and other regulators will be scrutinizing and examining your medical records during nearly every visit to your building. They will want to see that the medical records are up-to-date and accurately reflect the care being provided. Medical records that are unorganized or missing information can lead to further investigation and issues for the facility.

Documentation for the care being provided to the resident is also important for reimbursement. When a medical record is incomplete or pieces of the record are missing or are hard to find, this can result in inappropriate reimbursement.

HIPAA

Often, the medical records director serves as the facility's "privacy officer." This involves training staff on patient confidentiality matters and ensuring that privacy regulations are adhered to such as compliance with the Health Insurance Portability and Accountability Act (HIPAA).

One of the primary purposes of HIPAA is to protect private health information. The level of scrutiny surrounding patient confidentiality has been steadily increasing. In fact, regulatory bodies now conduct HIPAA-specific audits and surveys.

Aside from necessary business conversations at work, no staff member should ever under any circumstance discuss information such as residents who are admitted to or are receiving care at the facility, current medical condition, diagnosis, etc. HIPAA violations can result in huge penalties and fines and even jail time for willful perpetrators.

Protecting the private health information of all who enter your doors is critical, and the medical records department can play a key role in this regard.

Code Status

As mentioned in the previous chapter, one extremely important document in every SNF is the DNR form. It is critical that staff understands and follows residents' wishes in the event that they stop breathing. Resuscitation efforts can sometimes lead to lasting and permanent health consequences that greatly diminishes an individual's independence and quality of life.

The medical records director, often in conjunction with the admissions coordinator and the social services director, ensures that every patient has an updated code status with a completed DNR form and that this information is clearly communicated to all team members. This documentation is very important for knowing how to respond to a resident in the event of an emergency.

Conclusion

There are many regulations pertaining to medical records, such as how to handle records after a death, how long records must be retained, and how often records and systems must be reviewed by a medical records consultant. Like many regulations, these change often and vary by state. The medical records director should always keep current with the latest rules. Compliance will protect and safeguard the facility. Though often a medical records department is only made up of one or two individuals, their role is vital to running a successful operation.

KEY TAKEAWAYS

- When it comes to medical records, great organization is the key to success. Maintaining thorough and complete records is a must.
- Records may be requested for review at any time; thus they must always be up-to-date, accurate, and easy to retrieve.
- Protected health information must be kept confidential. Staff should be well-trained on HIPAA regulations and the importance of confidentiality.
- Poor recordkeeping can hurt a facility in many ways, including impacting the quality of care and the financial performance of a facility.

TASKS TO EXPAND YOUR LEARNING

- ☐ Do a chart audit with the medical records director on a new admit, a long-term resident, and a discharged resident.
- ☐ Review the most recent medical records consultant's report and discuss it with the medical records director.
- ☐ Learn what steps are taken with a resident's record if he or she passes away.

COMMON POSITIONS IN THE DEPARTMENT

Medical records director – Though the functions of a medical records director can vary by facility, this individual's main responsibility is ensuring that medical records are always orderly and complete. They respond to medical records requests in a timely manner and ensure that proper documentation is provided when needed. They attend meetings as necessary. They often serve as the facility's "privacy officer" and take the lead on compliance with confidentiality rules and regulations. The medical records director may also play a key role in interdepartmental communication, helping to make sure that everyone is aware of any critical changes to residents' medical needs.

Medical records assistant – Helps the medical records director as assigned. Many facilities do not have a need for an assistant.

Human Resources

Introduction

When I think of human resources (HR) in the context of a SNF, I think first and foremost of the all the critical people systems that have a huge impact on the facility's performance. These systems include the interview process, onboarding process, new employee orientation, performance reviews, recognition and rewards, and coaching and disciplining of staff. Though your HR director will be involved with these systems, successful administrators also take an active role in each of them.

The role of the administrator in each HR system varies among facilities. However, the more the administrator is involved (without creating a bottleneck), the better. In many ways, a facility's people systems hold the key to its culture and its overall employee experience. Because of this, it is important to often consider what it is like to interview, onboard, attend new employee orientation, etc., at your facility. If employee turnover is high and morale is low, addressing your people systems is a great starting point for focusing on improvement. One of the biggest mistakes administrators make is not being involved enough in their people systems.

Your HR director will have many duties, but their most important responsibility is overseeing and coordinating the people systems. It is important to understand that in most SNFs, HR directors do not have lots of HR experience or expertise, or even a degree in the field. Usually they are experienced payroll clerks or skilled receptionists with an interest in HR functions. This doesn't mean they can't add a lot of value or be a significant contributor to your facility. It only means they may need guidance and training from you on the more strategic functions of HR.

Good HR directors in SNFs see themselves as employee advocates and view staff as their primary customers. As they learn to make the employee experience their number-one priority, they can have a big impact on performance at the facility.

Three Regulatory Compliance Functions

In addition to coordinating and overseeing the people systems mentioned, there are several critical functions regarding regulatory compliance that are often handled by the HR director, depending on the facility. Let's take a look at them.

1. **Background checks.** Facilities must conduct initial background checks upon hire, plus annual follow-up background checks. There are certain crime convictions that can preclude individuals from working in a SNF, where many of the customers are vulnerable and can be easily taken advantage of. Making sure you aren't employing such individuals is important for the well-being of those you serve.

2. **Verifying and tracking staff licensing.** The HR director must ensure that employees are in good standing and do in fact have the credentials they claim to have, such as a nursing license or nursing aide certification. And most professionals with a license or certification are required to do some form of continuing education to keep their credentials active. It is critical for the HR director to make sure staff members keep up with their credentialing and remind them, if needed, to get it done.

3. **Personnel file maintenance.** Nearly every time a surveyor enters the facility's doors—and always during the annual survey process—he or she will look at some

personnel files. This is to ensure that essential tasks have been completed, such as skills checkoffs, background checks, license verifications, new employee orientations, etc. Maintaining organized and complete personnel files is a must for the HR director.

Other Duties

The HR director should also know the employee handbook well and offer insights, reminders, explanations, and trainings on its contents as needed.

Some additional important functions often handled by this leader in a SNF include offering guidance on employee benefits; handling and following up on workers' compensation claims; overseeing the onboarding process and the completion of new hire paperwork; helping to investigate sexual harassment, discrimination, and other employee concerns and complaints; coordinating annual performance reviews and employee satisfaction surveys; participating in unemployment-related tasks; keeping up with OSHA requirements and compliance; managing FMLA and other leaves of absence; tracking attendance of staff at meetings such as new employee orientation; and assisting with disciplinary actions, off-boarding, and terminations.

Discipline and Terminations

It's important for all administrators to keep an eye on the way staff members are treated by their supervisors. Studies have shown that most employees leave an organization because of their relationship with their direct supervisor. To ensure that everyone is being treated fairly, the administrator can reinforce the need to follow a progressive disciplinary track when disciplining team members.

A progressive disciplinary track uses specific disciplinary steps that give employees proper warning when they are not meeting expectations, and allows them a chance to improve. A progressive disciplinary track should be followed under most circumstances. However, there are circumstances that may lead to immediate termination, such as abuse.

A progressive disciplinary track commonly includes the following steps:

coaching → verbal warning → written warning → final written warning → termination

Coaching is an important step in this process because it allows a supervisor to help an employee make adjustments before formal discipline. Few people willfully make mistakes or try to do a bad job at work. Good administrators encourage supervisors to use opportunities to coach and retrain as often as possible.

In terms of disciplining your department heads, it is imperative to document important conversations you have with them regarding their performance. One effective way to do this is to send a follow-up email to the employee after the conversation summarizing the discussion and your expectations for them and their department moving forward. The purpose of this email is to provide clarity and reinforce what was discussed. It is also less threatening and more flexible than a formal disciplinary form but can serve as documentation if termination is eventually needed.

Remember, under the Equal Employment Opportunity Commission, it is against the law to discriminate against anyone based on their sex, race, religion, color, national origin, age, or physical or mental disabilities. You and your HR director should keep an eye out for this at your facility.

One final thought to consider: the way you handle disciplinary actions, including terminations, will have a big impact on the culture of your facility. Be kind, listen, and never rush through a disciplinary action or termination. Make sure you set aside ample time to give individuals the attention and respect they deserve. And always have another team member

present with you during formal disciplinary actions and
terminations. Often this person may be your HR director.

CHAPTER 11 SUMMARY

KEY TAKEAWAYS

- The HR director will have a big impact on the facility's workplace culture and overall employee experience.
- The HR director should view facility staff as their number-one customer and do all they can to serve them.
- The administrator should be closely involved in people systems such as the interview process and new employee orientation.
- Critical HR functions include background checks, licensure verification, and maintaining personnel files.
- The facility's workplace culture is affected by the way disciplinary actions, including terminations, are handled.

TASKS TO EXPAND YOUR LEARNING

- ☐ Do an employee file audit, run a background check, and verify a license.
- ☐ Review all of your people systems and ensure they are designed to help create the best employee experience possible.
- ☐ Analyze workers' compensation claims from the past year and look for any patterns. At the monthly all-staff meeting, make it a regular practice to discuss any employee injuries that occurred that month and go over ways to avoid similar incidents in the future.

COMMON POSITIONS IN THE DEPARTMENT

Human resources/payroll director – These two important roles are nearly always handled by the same person and sometimes this position may even include other duties such as processing accounts payable (we will talk about payroll in the next chapter and accounts payable in Chapter 23). This person oversees all HR aspects of the business, including the onboarding and off-boarding of staff members, maintaining personnel files, and offering expertise and assistance as needed for disciplinary actions and staff development.

CHAPTER 12

Payroll

Introduction

Payroll is nearly always handled by a facility's HR director, and it is an extremely important process for two reasons. First, wages typically account for roughly 65-70% of a facility's total expenditures, so errors, mismanagement, or carelessness around the payroll process can be costly and hurt financial performance. Second, payroll affects people's livelihoods. Mistakes can cause staff a great deal of stress, mistrust, and burden. The individual responsible for payroll must be organized and on the ball.

Labor Review

Verifying that payroll and labor hours are accurate is one of an administrator's most critical roles. Though not the most exciting task, and not the reason why anyone ever decided to become an administrator, monitoring labor on a daily basis is crucial. A lack of oversight can cost the facility thousands of dollars each month.

When monitoring hours daily, an administrator should look for a few things. First, did staff members clock in and out at the appropriate times? Often, staff will tend to clock in as soon as they arrive to work (even if they are 30 minutes early) and then clock out whenever they leave (which might be 15 minutes late as they wait for their ride or linger in the breakroom). These additional minutes before and after scheduled shifts are commonly referred to as "clock creep."

Using the examples above, let's assume a position is budgeted for an 8-hour shift, but the employee works 8 hours and 45 minutes because they are clocking in early and clocking out late. Added up, this puts the facility five hours over budget by the end of the week. Now imagine multiplying those five hours by 100 employees! The payroll director can help the administrator and department heads monitor clock creep and hold staff members accountable for following their schedules.

Another thing to look for while reviewing labor each day is did staff members clock out for their lunch break? Again, an 8-hour shift can turn into 8 ½ hours if a team member simply fails to clock out for lunch. This will put the facility 2 ½ hours over budget by the end of the week, assuming the employee works five days a week. As with clock creep, the payroll director can help the administrator and department heads monitor lunch breaks and reeducate staff as needed on proper procedures for clocking in and out during breaks.

The last thing to pay specific attention to during your daily labor review is overtime hours. Overtime can add up quickly and take you well over budget, so you should be aware of who is working overtime and who is approaching overtime. Based on your findings during your daily review, schedules can be adjusted and staff can be shifted around to minimize overtime hours. The goal should be that every staff member works the specified number of hours assigned to their position each week (or day, depending on your state's overtime rules) without going into overtime. Inevitably there will be times when employees need to work overtime to meet the needs of the customers, but not monitoring overtime closely will lead to unnecessary and avoidable spending.

It is common for the administrator to ask the payroll director to print out a report showing the previous day's hours worked by department and hand out copies to department heads in stand-up meetings. It is also common for the administrator to ask the payroll director to maintain a labor hours tracking spreadsheet so the administrator can easily view, assess, and monitor hours worked each day. These are among the payroll director's critical assignments.

Other Duties

One headache nearly every payroll director faces is dealing with time adjustment forms. These are forms staff members fill out when they forget to clock in or out at the beginning or end of their shift or for lunch breaks. The payroll director must then manually enter in the punches that were missed. This can be very time consuming and can lead to payroll errors. If an employee frequently submits time adjustment forms, the payroll director should notify the employee's supervisor so they can coach them on the importance of clocking in and out. If the problem persists, the supervisor may need to take further disciplinary action.

Often the payroll director monitors and tracks work attendance. They also make sure vacations, holidays, and sick days are paid appropriately. Remember, good payroll directors are sensitive to the burdens faced by staff and the facility when employee paychecks are not correct, and they do all they can to ensure accuracy.

SNFs sometimes struggle with payroll-related legal regulations, such as those pertaining to exempt and non-exempt status, staff members working off the clock, and state and federal overtime laws. It's important to familiarize yourself with these laws and ensure adherence in order to protect your facility.

KEY TAKEAWAYS

- At most facilities, wages make up over 65% of total dollars spent.
- Accurate payroll is very important to the staff and to the facility.
- Labor hours must be monitored *daily* by the administrator—this is one of their most critical roles. Not closely monitoring wages can cost the facility thousands of dollars a month.
- Clock creep, missed lunches, and overtime are the three biggest causes of extra wage spending and must be monitored closely.

TASKS TO EXPAND YOUR LEARNING

- ☐ Prepare payroll for a pay period and enter in time adjustments, vacations, holidays, etc.
- ☐ Become familiar with the facility's payroll processing systems and software. Learn how to pull important reports such as a detailed labor report and wages report.
- ☐ Determine the percentage of total wage expenditures to your total spending. Do your wages make up more or less than 65% of your total spend?
- ☐ Review the cost of wages in each department. Determine what percentage of your total wage expenditures are from each department.

□ Look at overtime trends. Is the facility improving its total dollars spent on overtime? Which department is spending the most on overtime?
□ Become closely familiar with your state's overtime laws.

COMMON POSITIONS IN THE DEPARTMENT

Payroll/human resources director – These two important roles are nearly always handled by the same person (see Chapter 11). This person oversees all payroll functions for the facility and ensures that the payroll processes and systems are in place. They help monitor overtime as well as the proper procedures for clocking in and out. They run reports, track hours worked, enter time adjustments, and keep supervisors apprised of staff members who are failing to clock in and out properly. They do all they can to make sure employee paychecks are always accurate.

CHAPTER 13

CNA Care

Introduction

It is hard not to argue that certified nursing assistants (CNAs) are the most important people at a skilled nursing facility. They interact more frequently with your customers on a daily basis than any other staff. Because of this, CNAs will largely determine the experience customers have at your facility. It is imperative that you employ the best CNAs and that you take great care of them.

Being a CNA is hard work—period. There is very little that is glamorous or easy about it. However, CNAs have a tremendous impact on the lives of those they serve, so the job can and should be very rewarding. Reminding your CNAs of this and applauding them for their efforts is a great way to engage them and earn their trust.

Most of a CNA's responsibilities revolve around residents' activities of daily living (ADLs). ADL care includes assisting with toileting, eating and drinking, dressing, grooming, ambulation, bed mobility, and personal hygiene. CNAs may also take on a wide range of other tasks, from attending activities with residents to occasional cleanup and housekeeping. Regardless of what their duties are, CNAs are doing hard work for much of their shift.

Reimbursement

Not only are CNAs the face of the facility to your residents, they also play a significant role in reimbursement. Medicare, Medicare replacement, and most state reimbursement programs pay the facility in part for the amount of ADL care provided to the resident. Therefore, it is critical that your CNAs understand how to appropriately document the care they provide. Frequent training and refreshers on proper ADL care documentation are a must.

Though there are many different ADLs that CNAs help with, there are currently only four that impact reimbursement. (This may change in the future with the introduction of different payment models.) These four ADLs—bed mobility, transfers, eating, and toileting—are known as the late loss ADLs. They are called late loss because they are typically the last activities people can do independently until they ultimately need assistance. It is critical to accurately document the amount of care provided for these late loss ADLs, since they impact reimbursement.

Let's define each late loss ADL very briefly.

Bed mobility is any movement that happens on the bed or mattress. It includes moving up or down in bed, sliding over on the mattress or turning side-to-side, sitting up in bed or moving to and from a lying position, or moving to the edge of the bed to transfer. The facility must document and take credit for any care provided in this regard.

Transfers involve moving a resident from one surface to another. Some examples include moving from the bed to a wheelchair, from a wheelchair to a dining room chair, or from a chair to a standing position. The facility should document and take credit for any transfer help staff provide to residents.

Eating is how the resident gets nutrition into their body, including nutritional intake by any means, such as a g-tube. Eating encompasses both food and drink. If staff help a resident by bringing a spoon to their mouth or by guiding a straw to their lips, they should document this and take credit for it.

Toileting includes using the restroom, commode, bedpan, urinal, etc., as well as changing a resident's briefs, transferring them from a wheelchair to a toilet, or emptying a bedpan. It also includes managing ostomies or catheter care, and helping to unzip, unbutton, or unbuckle clothing to allow the resident to use the restroom.

Remember, late loss ADL care is not only hard work—it is also important to the facility for reimbursement purposes. Your CNAs need to understand what each one of these ADLs means and how to appropriately document the level of care they provide. The facility's leadership team should help ensure that the CNAs take credit for their hard work.

Regulatory

The care provided by your facility's CNAs will be heavily scrutinized and observed during most regulatory visits, including the annual survey. This is another reason why your CNAs must be top-notch. The surveyors will want to watch a transfer using proper technique, observe the necessary infection control protocols, and see good incontinence care, among other typical CNA tasks and responsibilities. They will ask CNAs who the abuse prevention coordinator is, how to properly report abuse, and what to do in the event of an emergency such as a fire or a natural disaster. Making sure your CNAs are well-trained to provide excellent care not only enhances the quality of care, but also helps avoid negative outcomes during regulatory visits.

It can be a lot of pressure to provide care under the watchful eye of a surveyor. For this reason, CNAs should have someone observe their work on a regular basis so they can get used to it. These observations can be conducted by internal employees like the director of nursing, the assistant director of nursing, or other clinical leaders, or they can be conducted by external corporate nursing personnel. Regardless, practicing providing care while others are observing will help CNAs feel more confident when a surveyor comes to watch.

Communication and Customer Service

Communication between nurses and CNAs is also critical. For example, if a CNA observes something off or different about a resident, they need to report it to the nurse right away. Or if a nurse receives a physician's order that changes a resident's care needs, they need to let the CNAs know right away. Coordination and communication between these team members is so important to the overall quality of care the facility provides.

Customer service skills are also a must for CNAs. Training and teaching them on how to provide great customer service is essential.

Again, the experiences your residents have with CNAs will define their entire experience with your facility. Don't underestimate or devalue their importance in the success of your facility.

KEY TAKEAWAYS

- CNAs are the face of your facility to your customers. They have more interactions with your residents than any other team members. It is critical that they are well-trained and good at what they do.
- Proper documentation of late loss ADL care provided by CNAs is important not only for care purposes but also for reimbursement.
- CNA care is closely scrutinized and observed during annual surveys and most other regulatory visits.
- CNAs must be well-versed in how to provide great customer service.

TASKS TO EXPAND YOUR LEARNING

- ☐ Memorize the late loss ADLs and determine whether the CNAs at your facility are documenting them accurately.
- ☐ Find out how often the CNAs receive ADL training at the facility. Provide a training on the proper documentation of late loss ADLs.
- ☐ Observe the level of customer service being given by the CNAs. Provide a training on customer service based on your observations, both good and bad.
- ☐ Interview a few CNAs to find out how they became certified—what they had to do, what courses they had

to take, what tests they had to pass, and what they felt they learned during their CNA coursework.

☐ Interview a few residents to get their opinion on what makes a great CNA. Share your findings with the nursing leadership team as well as the CNAs.

COMMON POSITIONS IN THE DEPARTMENT

Certified nursing assistants (CNAs) – CNAs assist residents with their needs, including activities of daily living such as dressing, grooming, bathing, eating, and transferring. They work closely with the rest of the nursing team to identify and communicate changes in condition, well-being, and the overall health of the residents. They may assist with other duties, such as light housekeeping, trash removal, laundry, activities, etc. Documentation and customer service are also important parts of their responsibilities.

Restorative nursing assistants (RNAs) – RNAs are CNAs who are trained to help with restorative nursing programs, which are often designed or developed by a therapist and overseen by a licensed nurse. These programs may include activities related to assisted dining, communication, active or passive range of motion, toileting and/or bladder retraining, bed mobility, walking or transferring, and grooming. Documentation is an important part of restorative care.

Certified medication aides (CMAs) – Some states allow CNAs to become certified as CMAs, which allows them to administer certain medications. CMAs can reduce a nurse's workload when it comes to passing medications. Usually, a CMA's primary responsibility is to administer medications to residents throughout their shift.

CHAPTER 14

Nursing Care

Introduction

You may often hear that being a nurse isn't what it used to be. The tasks, duties, and responsibilities of a nurse have changed a lot over the years, and nurses have had to adjust to new ways of providing care and learn new skills to keep up.

Things That Have Not Changed

As much as things have changed, there are a few standard skills that will always be needed to provide quality nursing care. Similar to CNAs, good customer service is one of them. Good customer service is a key component to good nursing care. This has not changed. Nurses who demonstrate good listening skills, show compassion, and quickly respond to needs will greatly enhance the customer experience and satisfaction of their patients.

Another critical requirement for good nursing care that has not changed is the necessity for great communication and teamwork with coworkers and other health care personnel. This includes good communication and teamwork with CNAs, fellow nurses, and physicians.

Nurse communication with CNAs. The nurses at your facility are responsible for overseeing the work of the CNAs, and they must know what their CNAs are doing. Nurses should help prioritize CNAs' tasks and guide their work to meet the residents' needs. They must effectively communicate any changes of condition or changes to the plan of care for each resident.

Nurse communication with fellow nurses. Communication with other nurses is also very important. Between shifts, the outgoing nurse should give a thorough report (a verbal account of what took place during the shift, along with the status of each patient and any pending items that need to be addressed) to the oncoming nurse. Too often, critical information about patients is not passed on from one shift to the next, and important things get missed, resulting in poor care. Take a moment to re-read that sentence. It happens way too often in the skilled nursing setting. Poor handoffs during shift change can put the residents and the facility at high risk and may result in very negative outcomes. It is imperative your facility has strong systems in place to ensure seamless shift changes and excellent nurse-to-nurse communication.

Nurse communication with physicians. Finally, clear communication with physicians and other health care providers is a must. Just as the CNAs are the face of your facility to your residents, the nurses are the face of your facility to physicians. Your floor nurses have more interaction with physicians than anyone else at the facility.

Without a high level of communication and teamwork among your caregiving team, problems will arise. The key people in all of this communication and teamwork are your floor nurses.

One final important skill for providing high quality nursing care that has not changed is maintaining great communication with patients and their families. Before providing care, nurses should always tell a patient about what is going on and explain what they are doing. Nurses who communicate well with patients and families by following up timely and by keeping everyone informed of the care being provided along with any changes of condition will improve your facility's reputation. It is also important to note that skilled nursing facilities are required by law to inform the physician and family of any incidents, accidents, or changes in condition.

Things That Have Changed

Nurses are now required to document *a lot* these days—it has become a very big part of how they spend their time. Carefully describing incidents and events, the status and well-being of the patient, communications with physicians and families, and the care being provided by the facility is vital. Administrators and the nursing leadership team must review clinical documentation often and provide frequent training to nurses to improve their documentation skills. Poor or careless documentation can put the facility at high risk for tags, takebacks, lawsuits, complaints, and poor care.

The technical skills needed to care for nursing home residents has changed a lot. Your nurses' technical skills are very important and will determine the services you are able to provide to your customers. Being able to properly care for a wide variety of clinical needs will allow your facility to serve more people. Sicker patients with more complex needs are being pushed into the skilled nursing setting more than ever before, and this trend will continue. Enhancing nurses' knowledge and skills is an important function of the nursing leadership team and should be high on the list of priorities for most administrators. Facilities that are able to handle a wide range of care needs by improving their nurses' clinical capabilities will reap the benefits of a stronger census and a better reputation in the community. Investing in your nurses' skills will also build the competency and confidence of your team. Hospitals, physicians, and other health care partners are looking for SNFs that employ nurses with the skills needed to meet the needs of a sicker population.

More than ever before, nursing care and documentation is scrutinized closely. Whenever a surveyor comes to your facility, they will meticulously review documentation and nursing care. During the annual survey process, a surveyor will observe and evaluate the skills of your nurses, including wound care, g-tube care, IV care, and catheter care. The surveyors will also observe medication administration and will note the facility's medication error rate based on their observations. Just like CNAs, nurses should be comfortable with someone looking over their shoulder while they provide care.

Nursing and New Admissions

New admissions are the lifeblood of a facility, however they are very time-consuming for nurses. A new patient admission requires a lot of work, including many assessments and mounds of paperwork. Keeping your nurses motivated to welcome new residents with a smile and view them as a blessing, rather than as "more work," is a challenge for any leader. But it is an important task.

Good administrators understand how more admissions impact their nursing team and become savvy at keeping nurses excited about new admissions. Simple actions that can go a long way include surprising a nurse with dinner on a day busy with admissions or consistently expressing recognition and appreciation when admissions go well. Also, make sure that you and other members of your leadership team are always ready to assist your nurses when admissions are high. As the leader of the facility, rallying staff around new admissions and getting everyone to pitch in and help out will communicate that you are in this together. It will also show everyone just how important new admissions are to you and the facility.

Final Thoughts

Nurses tend to struggle more than other staff with following proper procedures for clocking in and out (i.e. when their shift is supposed to start and end, and for lunch). The truth is that nurses probably have the best excuse for their lack of compliance in this regard. Whether it's an admission that comes in at the end of a shift, an incident or accident that happens right at lunch break, or an upset physician or family member trying to get answers before the nurse's shift even begins, nurses can have a lot on their plate and often at the wrong times. Helping nurses understand how to work together, trust each other, and hand off tasks to colleagues (including to members of the nursing leadership team) can improve the likelihood that they will clock in and out properly. Nursing overtime is on the rise in the industry, and it costs a lot, so it can't simply be brushed aside. Good administrators and leaders find ways to help their nurses avoid unnecessary overtime while always encouraging them to provide a high level of care. Both can be done!

Providing nursing care in a SNF has changed a lot over the years and can be a pretty stressful and thankless job. Take good care of your nursing team—know them by name, check in with them frequently, offer to help, express appreciation, tell them often why their job is so important, and remind them of the difference they are making in people's lives. Being a nurse is a noble life calling and they need to be reminded of that often. Afterall your nurses, and CNAs for that matter, are taking care of others all day long but who is taking care of them? Hopefully it is you and the rest of your leadership team. Doing all of this for your nurses will really elevate the level of care provided at your facility because your nurses will know you care about them and recognize their work.

KEY TAKEAWAYS

- Good customer service and communication are important skills for nurses.
- Your nurses are the face of your facility to physicians and will greatly impact their perceptions of your facility.
- Documentation is a crucial part of a nurse's responsibilities. Nursing documentation is scrutinized often.
- Nursing care and documentation will be looked at closely during regulatory visits, including during annual surveys.
- An administrator must constantly work at helping nurses to always be excited about new admissions.
- The leadership team must take good care of their frontline caregivers at the facility.

TASKS TO EXPAND YOUR LEARNING

- ☐ Work side-by-side with a nurse as she or he handles a new resident admission. Learn exactly what is required of your caregiving staff upon admission.
- ☐ Observe the level of customer service being provided by the nurses, in particular to physicians and family members over the phone. Answer and handle a few calls that a nurse would typically take. Provide a customer service training to your nurses.
- ☐ Review several nurses' notes. Highlight examples of both good notes and bad notes in a training provided to

all the nurses. Recognize those who wrote the good notes shared during the training.

COMMON POSITIONS IN THE DEPARTMENT

LVN/LPN – These are nurses who completed a one-to-two-year program and whose scope and practice is different than that of an RN. Most of the skills and care required in SNFs can be accomplished by LVNs and LPNs. For this reason, it is common to find a lot more LVNs/LPNs than RNs in SNFs.

RNs – These are nurses who have completed a two-to-four-year program and have passed the NCLEX-RN exam. An RN can do everything that an LVN/LPN can, as well as many other nursing tasks. Because of their additional education and experience, RNs often have strong critical thinking skills and are better suited to work through complex problems and patient complaints.

Charge nurse/floor nurse – These can be either LVNs/LPNs or RNs. Their primary role is to oversee and provide care to a certain number of patients as assigned to them during their shift. They oversee CNAs, administer medications, do treatments, and provide other care functions according to the patient's plan of care. They also document care and patient status, communicate with physicians and families throughout their shift, and keep a close eye on any changes of condition in their patients. They complete admissions, discharges, and incidents as needed. They also give a thorough report to oncoming nurses to ensure there are no gaps in care.

CHAPTER 15

Nursing Administration

Introduction

The quality of nursing administration often makes or breaks a facility. As a SNF, the majority of your staff and the main services you provide fall under the responsibility of nursing administration. The nursing department also makes up a good portion of your total expenditures and overall budget. Because of all of this, the most critical role in your facility is the director of nursing (DON). The competence, confidence, and leadership of the DON will have a dramatic impact on your results.

The Administrator–DON Relationship

The relationship between the administrator and the DON is critical to a facility's success. A great administrator–DON partnership leads to good outcomes. When this relationship is strained or broken, the facility's success is jeopardized.

Like all relationships, it takes work, compromise, and a high level of communication for a strong administrator–DON relationship to exist. Setting expectations for your relationship from the very start and revisiting them often is what good partners do. Both the administrator and the DON should be comfortable sharing their opinions, disagreeing, and talking through differences with each other. These conversations should happen behind closed doors. When in front of others, the administrator and the DON should always present a united front.

Ultimately, you and your DON should have the same end goal. Keeping in mind the mission and vision of the facility will help you work through your differences.

Nursing Leadership

The quality of your assistant director of nursing (ADON) or unit managers (UMs) is also very critical. These leaders often have the most frequent interaction with your clinical staff. Since nursing is by far the biggest department in a SNF, the experience of most of your team will hinge on their interactions and relationships with the ADONs or UMs.

Your nursing leaders must be adept at training others. Much of what they do is review the work of the floor staff (nurses and CNAs) and provide training and education on nursing systems, documentation, and care. Being able to communicate well and hold people accountable in a positive way is important.

It's crucial for your nursing administration team to fully understand the facility's mission, vision, and values and the culture you are trying to build. As an administrator, you must do all you can to help the nursing leadership team to become role models and exemplify the culture you desire to have in your facility.

Nursing Leadership and Regulatory Visitors

The manner in which regulatory visitors perceive your nursing administration team will often influence your regulatory results. If the nursing leadership team seems caring, confident, and on top of things, surveyors will feel good about the quality of care being provided at your facility. If the nursing leadership team seems indifferent, rude, uncaring, and/or doesn't know the patients, families, and staff under them, the surveyors may consider it a red flag and look at your facility with a more critical eye. Great interpersonal skills—not only with staff, patients, and family members but also with regulatory visitors—are a must for all nursing leadership team members.

Other nursing leaders also play important roles at a SNF. In the Chapter Summary is a list of many of these roles and their responsibilities. We will talk in-depth about some of them in future chapters.

KEY TAKEAWAYS

- The DON is your most crucial team member and is critical to the success of the facility.
- The relationship between the administrator and the DON often mirrors the performance of the facility. Thus, a strong partnership is needed between these two key leaders, who should share the same end goal.
- The nursing leadership team largely dictates the experience the majority of your staff have at the facility—thus these team members must model the facility's culture.
- Survey outcomes are often skewed by the perception the surveyors have of your nursing leadership team.

TASKS TO EXPAND YOUR LEARNING

- ☐ Make a list of the facility's critical clinical systems. Then write down which team member is responsible for each system. Update this list frequently.
- ☐ Develop a plan to strengthen the administrator–DON relationship. Follow through with your plan.

COMMON POSITIONS IN THE DEPARTMENT

Director of nursing (DON) – The most critical role in the facility. Filling this position with the right person often goes hand-in-hand with the facility's success. The DON is the administrator's partner in ensuring that all aspects of the facility run well.

Specifically, the DON oversees the entire nursing department as well as the overall care provided at the facility. They supervise and manage other nurse leaders, clinical systems, staffing, budgets, and clinical outcomes. They foster and maintain important relationships with physicians, families, colleagues, and others. They help market and sell the facility as needed. The DON must be a strong and capable leader who is willing to talk through issues, compromise, problem solve with the administrator, and do all they can to help the facility be successful.

Assistant director of nursing (ADON) or unit manager (UM) – Assists the DON with their responsibilities, including overseeing clinical staff, systems, and care. If there is more than one ADON or UM, they often oversee a designated part of the facility as well as specific clinical systems. They attend important meetings, such as weekly standard of care meetings and monthly quality assurance and performance improvement meetings. They communicate frequently with staff, family members, and physicians and help problem-solve concerns. They help train staff and ensure that all clinical team members are aware of and are following the facility's care policies and procedures.

Director of staff development (DSD) – Oversees staff training and education. May help with staff scheduling. Ensures competencies are met and checked off. Provides initial orientations to new clinical team members. Works to continually improve the skill level of staff. Not all facilities have a DSD; many times these responsibilities are shared among the DON and ADONs.

Minimum Data Set (MDS) coordinator or nurse – Responsible for completing MDS assessments. Also often oversees and updates residents' clinical care plans, although at times this responsibility is given to ADONs or others. More information is provided about this role in Chapter 19.

Case manager – Helps oversee the relationship with community partners such as HMOs, MCOs, and other Medicare replacement programs, and communicates updates on care to them. Helps with discharge planning and often oversees a clinical system or two. Many facilities do not have a dedicated case manager, so these duties often belong to staff members, such as ADONs.

Wound nurse – Oversees the facility's entire skin system and program. Provides wound care and treatment to patients. Provides education to clinical staff, including CNAs, on proper skin care protocols, policies, and procedures, as well as how to avoid skin problems. Can also be responsible for other clinical systems, such as immunizations. Not all facilities have a dedicated wound nurse, in which case these duties are given to others.

Staffing coordinator – Oversees the scheduling of clinical staff. Ensures all staff is aware of their schedule, finds replacements when someone calls out, works the floor, and fills in as needed. Monitors and educates staff about overtime and proper procedures for clocking in and out. Often, this leader will have other duties and responsibilities, such as overseeing clinical systems and/or handling central supply and equipment. Not all facilities have a staffing coordinator, in which case these duties are given to other nursing leaders.

CHAPTER 16

Nursing Systems

Introduction

Nursing systems are at the heart of all a SNF does within its walls. These systems allow you to monitor important aspects of the care being provided to residents and also monitor their health and well-being. Strong clinical systems will lead to high-quality care and outcomes. And only by consistently producing high-quality outcomes will you be able to build your facility's reputation and gain long-term stability and success.

The most effective way for an administrator to oversee the facility's nursing systems and quality of care is to consistently attend clinical meetings.

Primary Clinical Systems

Typically, the DON and the nursing leadership team will divide up responsibilities for overseeing each different clinical system. Each individual leader monitors their assigned systems and reports on them during clinical meetings. Some of the most important clinical systems include skin, falls, weight loss/gain, restraints, antipsychotic medications, infection control, incidents and accidents, immunizations, and changes of condition. These major clinical systems may also be referred to as clinical subcommittees. Let's take a look at each.

Skin—This is perhaps the most important clinical system because of the risk and cost involved. Skin issues and facility-acquired pressure injuries (also known as pressure sores, pressure ulcers, or bed sores) are the leading cause of care complaints and lawsuits. Keeping your residents' skin healthy is important.

Skin is usually evaluated by CNAs during peri-care and bathing. Signs of redness or skin discoloration should be reported immediately to the nurse.

Pressure injuries develop when a person is unable to move (immobilization) or cannot understand that they must move (cognitive deficit) in order to relieve pressure on different parts of their body. Imagine lying in bed or sitting in a chair for hours without moving. This is what patients experience when the staff isn't vigilant about turning and repositioning. Inevitably, it leads to skin breakdown and pressure injuries. Certain chronic illnesses such as diabetes mellitus can also put someone at high risk for skin breakdown.

Pressure injuries most often occur on bony areas of the body, such as the tailbone, hips, shoulder blades, ankles, and heels. Poor nutrition and humidity can also increase the risk of developing pressure injuries. Pressure injuries are classified in four stages; the higher the number, the worse the injury. Some pressures injuries may also be classified as unstageable, meaning it isn't possible to determine an accurate stage at this point in time.

Even one facility-acquired pressure injury is too much and puts the resident's health and the facility at great risk. Closely monitoring the skin system should be a top priority for the administrator and the nursing administration team. Zero facility-acquired pressure injuries should always be the goal.

Falls—After pressure injuries, falls with injury are the next most common reason why people seek litigation against SNFs. Doing all you can to help residents avoid falls will allow you to provide good-quality care and avoid the high risk of injury associated with falling.

Falls can occur for numerous reasons. They are too often caused by external factors like poor lighting, tripping hazards (such as a call light cord on the floor), improper footwear, or slippery or wet floors. Other common reasons for falls include medications the patient is taking or cognitive deficits the patient may suffer from. Whatever the reason, utilizing and adhering to fall prevention interventions is a must.

Weight loss/gain—Helping patients maintain their weight is an important part of care. Gaining or losing too much weight can put them at risk for other health issues.

Weight change is considered significant when an individual loses or gains 5% of their weight in a 30-day timeframe, 7.5% of their weight in a 90-day timeframe, or 10% of their weight in a 180-day timeframe. Significant weight loss or gain is a sign that other health issues may be present. Monitoring and maintaining weight is a crucial aspect of providing high-quality care to the elderly.

Restraints—Restraints are devices used to restrict or limit an individual's movement. For the most part, SNFs strive to do all they can to avoid using restraints. However, they may be used when necessary and appropriate to maintain a resident's safety. It is important to understand that the use of restraints will nearly always be looked at extremely closely by surveyors.

To be in compliance with restraint use, you must have a physician order and consent from the family or resident. The restraint must be removed every two hours for 15 minutes; this must be monitored and documented. Also, the facility must actively seek alternatives to reduce or eliminate use of the restraint. Besides physical restraints, there are also chemical restraints, such as medications used to lessen an individual's activity.

Antipsychotic medications—In recent years, there has been a big push to reduce the use of antipsychotic medications in the SNF setting. Many antipsychotics have negative side effects, and at times are not effective. For this reason, facilities must keep a close eye on them and make efforts to lessen their use.

Most facilities have antipsychotic usage goals in which they aim to continually lower the percentage of residents using these medications. One important regulation to keep in mind is that there must be an appropriate diagnosis to justify antipsychotic medication use. Without a proper diagnosis, the facility opens itself up to a risky situation that can lead to regulatory tags or citations, fines, and other negative outcomes.

Infection control—For obvious reasons, controlling the spread of infection is paramount in any health care setting. Having protocols to prevent the spread of infection and ensuring staff members are adhering to them is critical. Proper handwashing is the number-one infection control method. Surveyors will pay close attention to handwashing during their visits.

Infections acquired by a patient while at the facility are called nosocomial infections. These infections are monitored closely and facilities must do all they can to prevent and eliminate them.

Incidents and accidents—Preventing incidents and accidents is often within a facility's control. Reviewing each one that occurs and discussing how to prevent similar occurrences should be an important part of the daily routine of the facility interdisciplinary team. Typically, an administrator must sign off on incident and accident reports to acknowledge that they are aware of them and that they agree with the measures taken to rectify the situation and prevent recurrence.

Immunizations—Immunizations are important to the health of both residents and staff. Properly offering and tracking immunizations will help the facility provide better care. Facilities are required to make certain immunizations, such as the flu vaccine, is available to residents and staff each year.

Change of condition—The change of condition system is perhaps the most important clinical system because it encompasses all of the others. A change of condition log tracks changes or events pertaining to a resident's care, such as new medication orders, falls, incidents or accidents, elevated temperature, lab results, and restraint use. Daily monitoring of changes of condition will help a facility continuously meet residents' needs and improve the quality of care. When changes of condition are not monitored on a daily basis, important clues about a resident's well-being may be missed, possibly resulting in poor outcomes and poor quality of care.

Clinical systems must be reviewed often. Typically, it is a good idea to have a daily clinical meeting or include a clinical portion on the agenda of your daily stand-up meeting. During this time, each system is quickly reviewed, especially the change of condition log. A more thorough and detailed review happens weekly during the standard of care meeting. At this meeting, each clinical subcommittee is reviewed, and discussions around each system, how to minimize negative outcomes, and how to improve results takes place.

The Quality Assurance and Performance Improvement (QAPI) committee must meet quarterly, and it must include the medical director, the DON, and at least three other members at a minimum. Though the regulation is to hold a quarterly meeting with these specific individuals in attendance, it is a best practice to have a monthly QAPI meeting with your medical director and the entire interdisciplinary team.

The QAPI meeting must also be an open meeting in which any staff members can participate. The day and time of the meeting should be posted in a prominent location, such as by the employee time clock.

In the meeting, you should discuss and review each clinical subcommittee and then make plans to improve where necessary. These plans are often referred to as PIPs (performance improvement plans), and they should be well-documented. During an annual survey, the survey team will review your QAPI system thoroughly. They will ask the administrator and the DON about the QAPI meeting process, as well as about which specific improvements have been made recently as a result of the process. It is important for the administrator to ensure that the QAPI system is working, and to be prepared to answer questions about it.

Other Clinical Systems

There are other clinical systems that aren't considered clinical subcommittees, per se, but are extremely important and may be reviewed in QAPI meetings—especially if there are problems with the system. They include the tracking of labs, x-rays, and pharmaceuticals. Failing to proactively communicate and respond quickly to issues around these systems can lead to some serious negative outcomes and quality-of-care issues.

A newer clinical system that is rapidly gaining attention and significance is the prevention of re-hospitalization. With reimbursement now tied to recidivism (sending a patient back to the hospital), SNFs are paying close attention to how to reduce re-hospitalizations. This emerging clinical system should be in place at every facility. It includes the monitoring, planning, and prevention of hospital readmissions (also known as "returns to acute," or RTAs). Working together to prevent unnecessary re-hospitalizations should be on your QAPI and standard of care meeting agendas. There are many tools the nursing team can use to better communicate with physicians when evaluating the needs of a resident.

One last longstanding clinical system is the 24-hour log. This is a helpful log that allows nurses to communicate what happened during their shift. In the event that something is missed during a verbal report between shift changes, the 24-hour log can be a safeguard, since it captures important information that takes places during each shift. Nurses should be trained to review the 24-hour log as soon as they begin their shift.

Again, clinical systems are at the heart of what we do in skilled nursing. Your team must be committed to and squarely focused on providing great care. If you hope to run a facility that sees strong and sustained results, you must provide good-quality care, period. And good-quality care starts with good clinical systems.

KEY TAKEAWAYS

- Having good nursing systems in place will improve the quality of care, which can lead to good long-term results.
- The best way for an administrator to oversee the facility's quality of care is by consistently attending clinical meetings.
- Major clinical systems or clinical subcommittees include skin, falls, weight loss/gain, restraints, antipsychotic medications, infection control, incidents and accidents, immunizations, and change of condition.
- The change of condition system is perhaps the most important of all because it encompasses all of the other systems and helps the facility quickly respond to changes any resident may experience.
- Clinical systems are reviewed and monitored in a daily clinical meeting or in the clinical portion of a daily stand-up meeting, weekly in a standard of care meeting, and monthly in a QAPI meeting.
- The QAPI meeting must include the medical Director, DON, and three other members, per the regulation. The administrator and the DON will be asked about the QAPI meeting and process during every annual survey.

TASKS TO EXPAND YOUR LEARNING

☐ In terms of improving care, what are your facility's clinical goals? Create a simple way to track and monitor progress toward those clinical goals.

☐ Make a list of all the clinical systems and who is responsible for each. Communicate this information with your entire leadership team so that everyone is clear on who has responsibility for each system.

☐ Spend a few hours monitoring handwashing in the facility. Report your findings to the staff and provide a training on the importance of proper handwashing.

☐ Review the lab and x-ray system in the facility. How are results communicated from the lab or x-ray company to the facility, from the facility nurses to the nursing leadership team, and from the facility to physicians? Determine if your current system is working well and make improvements if needed.

☐ Review the last three items that have gone through a PIP in your facility based on your QAPI process. Were the plans developed by the QAPI committee effective? Take the opportunity to complete the PIP form during the next QAPI meeting.

COMMON POSITIONS IN THE DEPARTMENT

The nursing administration team, including the DON, ADONs, UMs, DSD, wound nurse, case manager, MDS coordinator, etc., all typically help with upkeep, monitoring, and reporting regarding the important clinical systems. It is critical that the ownership of each system as well as its related responsibilities are clear to each leader. If a clinical system slips through the cracks and is not being monitored, bad things can happen.

Regulatory Basics

Introduction

A SNF holds a license that allows it to participate in Medicare and Medicaid programs. In order to keep this license and remain in good standing, the facility must adhere to all the rules and regulations surrounding the Medicare and Medicaid programs, which include both federal and state laws. When a facility fails to meet these rules and regulations, it can be cited for failure to do so. These citations for deficient practices are often referred to as tags. A facility risks losing its license if it continues to receive tags and fails to get back into compliance.

2567 Form

At the end of a visit by a surveyor, a facility is typically given an initial findings or observations form which may include a list of resident charts the surveyor looked at. Sometime after the visit, a 2567 form, also known as a Plan of Correction (POC) form, is sent to the facility. This usually happens via email to the administrator or DON. This form outlines the final observations and findings of the surveyor, and in the case of a citation, it explains how the facility failed to comply with a certain regulation. (If nothing was cited, the form will be blank.) The surveyor's findings are noted on the left side of the 2567 form. The right side of the form is blank when received by the facility. This is the space where the facility must write out its plan to correct the deficient practice. The state has 10 business days to send the 2567 form to the facility, and the facility has 10 calendar days to return the form (including the plan) to the state.

Once the completed 2567 form is submitted to the state, the state will either approve the plan or ask for changes or additional information—in which case the facility will need to rework its plan and resubmit it, repeating the process as needed until it is approved.

Once the plan is approved, the state will either conduct a desk review (essentially confirming that the submitted plan was reviewed and meets the requirements to get back into compliance), or send surveyors to the facility to ensure the plan is being followed as outlined in the 2567. If a facility continues to receive tags or fails to clear the tags they have received, it risks losing its license and therefore becoming ineligible to participate in Medicare and Medicaid programs. Fines known as civil monetary penalties (CMPs) can also be given by the state as a consequence for tags. More severe or repetitive tags (i.e. the facility has been cited for the same issue in the past) will result in higher CMPs.

2567 forms must be made available to the public by the facility. Many facilities keep a binder of these forms in the lobby. 2567 forms, including citations and tags, are also made publicly available online. Thus, the best way to safeguard your facility's reputation is by doing all you can to provide great care and avoid tags.

Tags

Not all tags are created equal. Tags are designated with letters from A through L. "A" is the lowest-level tag; "L" is the highest-level tag. In addition to the letter assigned to a tag, a citation can also be designated as a substandard quality of care (SQC) tag, which puts a spotlight on poor care. Tags with an SQC designation are more severe or serious than tags without it. This designation is related to tags within three deficient practice categories: 1) resident behavior and nursing home practices, 2) quality of life, and 3) quality of care. An SQC designation can be given to tags at an F level and above.

Below is what is known as the Scope and Severity Grid, which breaks down the different tag levels.

Health Inspection
Scope and Severity Grid

Severity	Scope		
	Isolated	Pattern	Widespread
Immediate jeopardy to resident health or safety	J	K	L
Actual harm that is not immediate jeopardy	G	H	I
No actual harm with potential for more than minimal harm that is not immediate jeopardy	D	E	F
No actual harm with potential for minimal harm	A	B	C

The *scope* refers to the number of residents impacted by the alleged deficient practice, and the *severity* is the seriousness of the problem and its potential to cause harm.

Tags can be issued at any given moment during any visit by a surveyor and can potentially have huge ramifications on the facility. Surveyors may enter your building at any time and review the practices of the facility to make sure all rules and regulations are being followed. The most common types of visits include the annual survey (also known as a fullbook survey) and complaint and self-report visits. These are described below.

Annual Survey

Annual surveys are supposed to happen once a year and should take place between 9 and 15 months from the last annual survey. (A few states struggle to complete all of their annual surveys timely.) This 9-to-15-month timeframe is commonly referred to as the fullbook survey window.

The annual survey includes two different kinds of surveys: the health survey and fire safety survey. The health survey addresses compliance with all the health rules and regulations, while the fire safety survey focuses on fire-safety codes and regulations. There is some overlap between these two sets of rules and regulations, but generally the health survey focuses on the care and services being provided while the fire safety survey focuses on the accessibility and safety of the building.

Many predictable things happen during the annual survey. For example, medication administration, wound care, transfers, and peri-care will be observed. Surveyors will inspect the laundry room and kitchen. Meal service will also be watched. A surveyor will attend and ask questions to residents during a resident council meeting.

Additionally, staff will be questioned about the proper way to report abuse. Recent self-reports—specifically those about abuse—will be reviewed. The surveyors will always ask to see the abuse policy, including investigation procedures when abuse is reported or suspected, and may ask staff about it. The surveyors will also interview the administrator about abuse prevention as well as the QAPI program. In terms of the QAPI program, the surveyor will want to know about recent problems that were identified and improved by the facility as a result of its QAPI process.

Complaint and Self-Report Visits

Surveyors may visit your facility based on a complaint they received about your facility or a self-report. (A self-report is when a facility reports itself to the state.) A self-report is required to be submitted to the state by the facility for serious incidents such as the elopement of a resident or an allegation of abuse. Each state has its own specific rules and regulations surrounding self-reports. Failing to self-report appropriately can lead to tags and further investigations.

Complaint and self-report visits can happen at any time. These visits are prioritized by the perceived severity of the complaint or self-report. Those that seem to have potential for harm if not addressed immediately will be prioritized and will trigger an immediate visit by a surveyor. If complaints or self-reports do not seem very serious, a surveyor may not visit the facility for many days, weeks, or possibly months. Any outstanding self-reports or complaints will normally be handled during the annual survey if they have not already been looked at. Also note that self-reports or complaints previously investigated can be reviewed and investigated again by the annual survey team.

Surveyors

It is important for all staff to know that a surveyor's job is to investigate, inspect, and write tags when deficient practices exist. Different surveyors take different approaches to the investigation process. Whether their approach is friendly and talkative or rude and pushy, it is imperative to understand that all surveyors are at your facility for the same reason. It is just as possible for a friendly surveyor to give you lots of tags, as it is for a rude surveyor to give you none.

Staff should not panic when surveyors are in the building. They should be trained on how to work with and talk to surveyors, and they should know to always be concise and truthful in their answers to surveyors' questions. Sharing assumptions, perceptions, or information that is not requested should be avoided, as it may lead to further investigations and citations. Remind staff often to share only what they know to be facts and only the information requested. And if they don't know the answer to something they should answer truthfully and offer to find out the answer. Never should a staff member take a guess about something they may not know. Educating and preparing staff for surveyor visits is an important responsibility of the administrator and the DON.

Regulatory Success

The key to regulatory success is to be *survey ready* every hour of every day. Too often facilities take it easy when they are not in the annual survey window and then ramp things up when in the window. This creates bad habits and practices, which opens the door for mistakes and tags. You and your team should always be doing the right things in the right ways. Accountability and high standards must always be in place regardless of the expected timeframe for the annual survey. Facilities should be ready at any given moment to impress a surveyor. After all, they can walk into the building at any time.

Building relationships with the local department of health is a good idea for an administrator. Upon starting at a new facility, you should always try to schedule an in-person meeting with the program manager (the leader who supervises the surveyors in the area—this person can have different titles in each state) to introduce yourself and share your vision and passion for the facility. This is also a great time to learn anything you can about the history of the building and the perception of the building from a regulatory standpoint.

After this initial visit, when questions arise about regulatory matters, a wise administrator will reach out to and touch base with the program manager to further develop the relationship and get their thoughts and opinions. Many program mangers enjoy the opportunity to educate administrators working in their region.

Another reason for having a good relationship with the program manager is if something does go wrong at your facility, the program manager will know the building is led by someone who is caring, committed, and competent. This will go a long way in reassuring the regulatory team that the incident was an unusual occurrence rather than willful carelessness. Without an established relationship, it is easy for a program manager and surveyors to assume the worst about an administrator when something negative happens at a facility. Thus, finding ways to communicate with the program manager on a fairly consistent basis to build a relationship is a very good idea.

Ombudsperson

Finally, the ombudsperson can be a big help to your facility. They work for the state, though they are not a surveyor and they do not write tags. The ombudsperson is assigned to multiple SNFs in a designated area. Their primary function is to help advocate for the residents.

Typically, an ombudsperson is well-versed in rules and regulations and understands the challenges SNF operators often face in caring for the elderly population. This person can provide insight, ideas, and assistance in difficult situations. They can talk to families and residents and help explain rules, regulations, and reasonable expectations.

If you develop a strong relationship with the ombudsperson, they can become a huge advocate for your facility and can help you quickly resolve even the toughest of situations. Surveyors love it when a facility involves the ombudsperson in sticky and difficult situations. It is advantageous for administrators to lean on and fully utilize the expertise of the ombudsperson assigned to the facility.

CHAPTER 17 SUMMARY

KEY TAKEAWAYS

- It is imperative to stay in good standing and protect the facility's license by avoiding tags (citations for deficient practices).
- Surveyors can enter a facility and start an investigation at any time.
- Tags can have significant ramifications on the facility.
- Good administrators ensure that their facility is always survey-ready. They also develop relationships of trust with their local program manager and facility ombudsperson.

TASKS TO EXPAND YOUR LEARNING

- ☐ Make an annual survey preparation binder that includes information the survey team will want upon arrival.
- ☐ Review the observations and findings on the 2567 form from the most recent annual survey. What was the facility cited for? Review the facility's submitted plan of correction and ensure the plan is still in place.
- ☐ Contact the program manager and schedule an in-person meeting. Introduce yourself and ask about the survey process in the area. Specifically ask about when a facility should and should not self-report certain incidents.
- ☐ Contact the ombudsperson and schedule an in-person meeting. Find out how they feel about your facility and

what they believe is your biggest opportunity to improve it.

PEOPLE YOU SHOULD KNOW

Program manager (also known as a program director, or may have a different title depending on the state) – This person leads and directs state surveyors within a geographic area in the state. A program manager will be assigned to your facility and oversees the survey activity that happens there. This person carries a lot of influence and can directly impact the regulatory outcomes at your facility. Administrators must get to know their program manager and strive to work effectively with them.

Ombudsperson – Every state is required under the federal Older Americans Act to have an ombudsperson program. An ombudsperson addresses complaints and advocates for residents in an assigned area. This includes helping the elderly in SNFs, assisted living facilities, and other similar adult care facilities. An ombudsperson is trained to resolve problems and work with all parties involved to come to the best resolutions possible. An ombudsperson may be a volunteer or a paid employee of a state government agency. It is important for the facility to have a strong relationship with this person.

CHAPTER 18

CMS Star Rating

Introduction

The Centers for Medicare & Medicaid Services (CMS) Five-Star Quality Rating System is ever changing and evolving, and administrators can expect more variations in the future. In fact, depending on when you read this book, it is highly possible that some of the information provided here has already changed.

Most importantly, administrators must understand that a facility's CMS star rating is significant and can have a big impact on business. However, a low star rating doesn't mean that a facility can't become highly successful. Administrators should know that with the right focus and the right strategies in place, the rating of their facility can improve quicker than they might realize.

Impact on Business

CMS star ratings are available to the public. Whether fair or not, it is inevitable that some people will use your star rating to determine the quality of your facility. This rating has the potential to affect your facility's reputation and hurt or help your ability to attract new clients and staff. The truth is, more and more people are becoming aware of the star-rating system and are using it as a primary decision-maker when deciding where to send their loved ones or where to work.

Many potentially advantageous partners won't do business with a facility if its star rating is too low. For example, many HMOs, ACOs, and other alternative payers will only do business with facilities that meet certain established star-rating criteria. The star-rating system has made it easy for these providers to narrow their networks and minimize and control their partnerships with a limited number of SNFs. This has the potential to greatly impact a facility's ability to accept patients who have benefits within these networks. If there is a prominent ACO forming in your area, for instance, and it requires facilities to have at least a 4-star rating to be included in their network, yours may be out of luck if its rating is below that threshold.

How it Works

The CMS star-rating system can be confusing. It is composed of three domains: 1) health inspections, 2) staffing, and 3) quality of care measures. Not all of the domains are weighted equally. Each domain is awarded a star rating from 1 to 5, and together they make up the overall star rating. Let's take a quick look at each domain.

Health Inspections

The health inspections domain is based on the number of tags a facility has received over the past three years (though periodically it has changed between two and three years). This includes any tags received during the annual survey as well as during any other visits, such as a complaint visit. The star rating **does not** include any fire safety tags received by the facility— only health survey tags.

The health inspections domain incorporates a points system with more severe tags weighted greater than less severe tags. For example, A, B, and C level tags are 0 points (they don't negatively impact your star rating at all), a D level tag is 4 points, an E level tag is 8 points, and so on.

Health Inspection Score

Weights for Different Types of Deficiencies

Severity	Scope		
	Isolated	Pattern	Widespread
Immediate jeopardy to resident health or safety	J 50 points *75 points	K 100 points *125 points	L 150 points *175 points
Actual harm that is not immediate jeopardy	G 20 points	H 35 points *40 points	I 45 points *50 points
No actual harm with potential for more than minimal harm that is not immediate jeopardy	D 4 points	E 8 points	F 16 points *20 points
No actual harm with potential for minimal harm	A 0 points	B 0 points	C 0 points

Note: * indicates points for deficiencies that are for substandard quality of care

Once the points are added up, the star rating assigned to the health inspections domain is calculated based on a bell curve-like system for each state. What this means is a predetermined percentage of facilities in a given state will receive a 5-, 4-, 3-, 2-, and 1-star rating in this domain. So, the top 10% of the facilities with the fewest point totals are given a 5-star rating, the next 70% of facilities with the next fewest points are given 4-, 3-, and 2-star ratings, and the bottom 20% of facilities with the most points are given a 1-star rating. This means a facility can gain or lose a star in this specific domain without any surveys or tags causing the change—the change is simply due to the performance of other SNFs in the state. This domain carries the most weight in determining a facility's overall CMS star rating.

Staffing

Not too long ago, providers and facilities self-reported their staffing levels during annual surveys. However, that has recently changed. Payroll-based journaling (affectionately known as PBJ) has been rolled out by the government and is now used to track staffing for facilities. A facility's star rating for the staffing domain is based on the number of hours worked by licensed clinical staff in your building and is adjusted for case mix (your Resource Utilization Group [RUG] levels—i.e. higher RUG levels indicate a need for more staff, lower RUG levels indicate a need for less staff). A facility is also penalized for consecutive days without an RN working at the facility.

Essentially—or in theory, anyway—the more staff you have working, the higher your star rating will be for this domain. The fewer you have working, the lower the rating. If your staffing domain earns four or five stars, your overall star rating can gain a star. And if it earns one star, your overall star rating will lose a star.

Quality of Care Measures

The quality of care measures (QMs) domain has seen frequent adjustments to how its star rating is calculated. This domain's impact on a facility's overall star rating is very similar to the impact of the staffing domain. Earning five stars in the QMs domain will add one star to your facility's overall star rating, and earning one star will take away a star from the overall rating. Thus, QMs like staffing become super important, as they can boost or reduce your overall rating.

There are 16 QMs (for now) that impact a facility's star rating. They are divided between the common subpopulations of residents in a facility: short-stay and long-stay residents. These 16 QMs are:

<u>Short-stay residents</u>

1) Percentage of short-stay residents who were re-hospitalized after a nursing home admission

2) Percentage of short-stay residents who have had an outpatient emergency department visit

3) Percentage of short-stay residents who got antipsychotic medication for the first time

4) Percentage of short-stay residents with pressure injuries that are new or worsened

5) Percentage of short-stay residents who report moderate to severe pain

6) Rate of successful return to home and community from a short stay

7) Percentage of short-stay residents who improved in their ability to move around on their own

<u>Long-stay residents</u>

8) Percentage of long-stay residents who got an antipsychotic medication

9) Percentage of long-stay residents experiencing one or more falls with major injury

10) Percentage of long-stay residents with pressure injuries

11) Percentage of long-stay residents with a urinary tract infection

12) Percentage of long-stay residents who have or had a catheter inserted and left in their bladder

13) Percentage of long-stay residents whose ability to move independently worsened

14) Percentage of long-stay residents whose need for help with daily activities has increased

15) Percentage of long-stay residents who were physically restrained

16) Percentage of long-stay residents who report moderate to severe pain

The QMs, in theory, are an indication of the quality of care provided at your facility. This is yet another reason why the clinical systems talked about in Chapter 16 are so important to monitor because they can also help improve your QMs. (And as a side note, a facility's QMs also trigger surveyors on what to look for during the annual survey process.) You should also remember that not all QMs impact your star rating, only the 16 above (as of this writing).

In summary, the calculation of your overall CMS star rating starts with the health inspection rating. This rating is added to, left alone, or subtracted from based on the staffing and quality of care measures star rating. The remaining total stars are your facility's overall star rating.

Bad Star Rating
So, what if your facility's star rating is bad? Are you doomed to fail? Of course not! There are some steps you can take to minimize the impact and improve your rating. Let's look at a few.

First: if there is a portion of your star rating that is good, highlight that part of your rating and come up with ways to show off its importance. For example, if the QM domain earned a 5-star rating but health inspections and staffing only earned one star, you can make it known that the QMs are the best measurement for quality. Here are some facts you might highlight in this case:

1) The QM domain rating is the best indicator of quality of care because it looks at care over a prolonged period of time.
2) The health inspection domain rating is based on a single point in time at the facility, and includes subjective measuring.
3) The QMs are objective and are based on true outcomes over an extended timeframe.

This is a simple example of how you can strategize to create a message that will best help the facility. Focusing on what your facility is doing well and why it matters is one way to minimize the potential negative impact of a poor overall star rating.

Second: take credit for your staffing. Too often facilities fail to acknowledge and document hours worked at the building. Contractors, registry or agency staff, and even salaried employees are often forgotten. And what about that corporate nurse who was at your building helping your clinical team for a few days last week? Or the corporate MDS nurse who will be at your facility next week? Will you take credit for these people? Capturing all the hours people are working at your facility is so important. Own this domain by ensuring that every single hour worked by licensed personnel is accounted for, and your staffing star rating will improve.

Third: QMs are more within your control than you might think. A facility's QM information is derived from what the facility submits on the MDS. Too often, facilities carelessly document on the MDS and simply focus on completing the task rather than paying close attention to what is going on and accurately documenting it. Just because a patient has had a certain diagnosis in the past, or has had pain, or a wound, as some examples, doesn't mean they still do. Being vigilant about documentation—especially around those QMs that impact your star rating—is crucial.

Additionally, figure out and review which QMs your facility is struggling with and focus on those specific areas to improve care. Many facilities have greatly improved their QMs quickly by tightening up their documentation and systems and by focusing on improving care in the areas that most impact their quality of care measures star rating.

Fourth: always be survey-ready. Surveyors can walk through your door at any given time, so make sure your team is always doing the right things no matter what. Good habits lead to good survey outcomes, whereas bad habits can be hard to hide when it matters most. If you train your staff to know how to respond to and handle surveyors, and your always providing great care, your health inspection star rating will improve.

Star Rating Summary

At the end of the day, your facility has a big impact on its CMS star rating. Staffing appropriately and making sure to take credit for all hours worked, being attentive to QMs, and always being survey-ready will help you work your way to a great—and sustained—overall star rating. Good administrators begin improving their facility's star rating almost immediately by taking the actions described above.

The importance and impact of the CMS star rating will only continue to grow. And yes, it's true that the star-rating system is flawed and doesn't necessarily reflect the true quality of care at a facility. However, SNFs that embrace the system for what it is and choose to accept there are many things they can do to impact and improve their rating will come out on top.

KEY TAKEAWAYS

- The CMS star rating is becoming more and more important for facilities. Many providers will no longer do business with facilities that have poor star ratings, and the public is increasingly becoming aware of these ratings.
- The overall star rating is made up of three domains: health inspections, staffing, and quality of care measures.
- The health inspections domain is based on tags received during the last three years.
- The staffing domain only takes licensed staff hours worked into consideration and is adjusted for case mix.
- The staffing and quality of care measures domains can add or subtract from your overall star rating based on results.
- An administrator can take several immediate actions to impact their facility's star rating.

TASKS TO EXPAND YOUR LEARNING

- ☐ Evaluate your facility's current star rating. What is the overall star rating? What is the star rating for each different domain? Which domain's rating should you be highlighting to the public?
- ☐ Look up the five nearest competitors' star ratings to see where your facility stands in the local community.
- ☐ Figure out what your QM points currently are and how many points you need in order to earn five stars in this

domain. Review the 16 QMs that impact star rating and determine which are hurting you the most. Develop plans to improve in those areas.

☐ Do a comprehensive review of all of your clinical staff who work in the building to ensure you are taking credit for all hours worked.

CHAPTER 19

Revenue and MDS

Introduction

Reimbursement systems can be very confusing, and they take time to learn. Don't get too frustrated if you don't understand a reimbursement model right away. Make a commitment to studying and learning reimbursement systems over time.

There are two ways to improve a facility's financial performance: increasing revenue and cutting expenses. Successful administrators pull on the right levers for both. In this chapter, we will focus our attention on growing revenue. (Note: if there are acronyms in this chapter that you are not familiar with, please refer back to the common acronym guide in Chapter 3.)

Payer Sources

To begin, let's take a look at the major payer sources, including private pay, hospice, Medicaid, Medicare Part A, Medicare Part B, HMO and Medicare Replacement plans, and talk briefly about how each pays.

Private Pay

Typically, a facility will have one rate for a private room and a different rate for a semi-private room. Some facilities choose to have different levels of private payment based on care provided to the resident however this can be a lot of work. Most stick with just one rate for a private room and another for a semi-private room.

Private pay rates can vary quite a bit from facility to facility. It is also common for facilities to annually increase private pay rates (similar to the annual increase in Medicare copayments) to help keep up with inflation and the increasing costs of services and supplies. Private payers aren't normally your best payers, but they aren't usually the worst either.

Hospice
A patient can be in your facility and also be on hospice services. When this happens, the hospice company is responsible for paying the facility. Typically, the hospice company will pay the state Medicaid rate, although hospice contracts can be negotiated.

Medicaid
Reimbursement for Medicaid varies a lot by state in both the dollar amount and the payment model methods used to determine reimbursement. For many states, a RUG system is used. Although many states still use RUG-III, plenty of others utilize RUG-IV. With the introduction of the Medicare Patient-Driven Payment Model (PDPM), some states may choose to adopt a similar payment model soon.

No matter the Medicaid payment system, it is important to take time to learn as much as you can about your state's reimbursement system, with the goal of eventually having a thorough understanding of how your state reimburses for residents covered by Medicaid.

Medicare Part A
Medicare Part A provides short-term care coverage in a SNF (further explanation will be provided in Chapter 20). As of this writing, Medicare reimbursements are based on the RUG-IV system, though new payment systems are being developed and a change to the Patient-Driven Payment Model (PDPM) is slated for October 2019. RUG-IV consists of 66 categories or RUG levels which represent different payment amounts based on the documented services provided to the resident. The new PDPM system will be very different than the current RUG-IV system, as clinical services will take a more prominent role, changing from therapy minutes as the basis of payment. Regardless of the payment model, understanding what triggers reimbursement

and capturing all the services provided to the resident is key to reimbursement success.

HMO Payers or Medicare Replacement Plans

Like Medicare, Medicare replacement plans provide coverage for short-term benefits only and will not cover long-term care services (further explanation will be provided in Chapter 20). These payers traditionally pay in a few different ways. Some may pay based on the current Medicare payment system, while others will pay per a contracted rate. For those that pay per a contracted rate, some will have a single rate while others will have a few different levels of reimbursement based on the services being provided. Becoming familiar with your different HMO contracts and negotiating the correct level of reimbursement per the contract where applicable is very important.

Medicare Part B

Medicare Part B insurance covers outpatient services whereas Medicare Part A insurance covers in-patient services. At times, long-term care residents need some additional outpatient services that the facility can provide in order to help them maintain their highest level of functioning and independence. One very typical example of this is therapy services. If a long-term resident has Medicaid as their primary insurance, then the facility would be paid by Medicaid for room and board and basic services provided, and Medicare Part B would pay for the outpatient services or in this case, specifically, the therapy services. One important item to remember here is that providing therapy services to long-term care residents who truly need it not only generates Part B revenue but can often increase the Medicaid RUG level for reimbursement (in those states that use a RUG reimbursement system).

There are other items and services covered by Medicare Part B that can be billed by the facility, such as certain immunizations, insulin, and even some wound care products. Understanding how and when Part B insurance can be billed for

136

services is important for taking full advantage of your revenue opportunities.

Other Types of Payers

There are other contracts and alternative payers that your facility may obtain, such as a VA contract. Often these contracts are exclusive and vary widely by facility.

At the heart of most reimbursement models is clinical documentation. SNFs must take credit for all of the work and services they are providing to their residents in order to receive full reimbursement. Often dollars are left on the table by poor documentation and a lack of vigilance in capturing all the facility is doing to care for their customers.

The MDS Assessment and RUGs

The MDS assessment determines the reimbursement amount received by the facility for nearly every payer source. The MDS assessment consists of a significant amount of information about each resident and the care they are receiving, such as their diagnoses, the amount of therapy minutes received, and the amount of ADL assistance received. MDS nurses gather the information from the clinical records and complete the MDS assessment based on what they find in the clinical record. If information is missing from the clinical record, it can't be claimed on the MDS. Documentation must be present to always support what is inputted into the MDS assessment.

Most buildings have at least one dedicated MDS nurse (sometimes called an MDS coordinator) who is responsible for the completion of the MDS assessments—and who, in a very real way, captures your revenue. These nurses should spend time with patients and staff to ensure that the MDS assessments accurately reflect the needs of the residents and the care being provided. The MDS nurse should meticulously go through each clinical record to portray a true picture of all the needs of the resident and all the services provided to them by the facility. Where documentation is missing, confusing, or incomplete, the MDS nurse can also write nurse notes on observations they've made in order to solidify and clarify documentation. Additionally, they can ask the nurses and CNAs caring for the resident to add additional documentation to more clearly paint a picture of the resident's needs.

The current RUG-IV system for Medicare reimbursement is going away very soon. However, a discussion about RUGs is still relevant, as many state Medicaid programs will continue to pay based on a RUG system. Additionally, as things stand right now, RUGs will play a factor in the nursing component of PDPM—though not as prominent a role.

A RUG is made up of a combination of three letters and numbers. Each letter and number represents something about the care being provided to the resident. The information entered into the MDS assessment determines the RUG level, and the RUG level—based on the current payment models—determines your reimbursement.

The assessment reference date (ARD) is the date a facility selects to base the assessment on. For example, if a facility choses November 30th as the ARD, then all of the information provided will be generated from that specific day. Selecting the ARD that best captures the services you are providing to a resident is important for reimbursement.

Let me reiterate the importance of selecting the most favorable ARD. Everything provided in the MDS assessment is based on the specific ARD. For example, if a facility completes providing seven days of breathing treatments today but has selected the ARD to be three days ago, they will not be able to claim all seven days of that service on the MDS assessment because some treatments happened after the ARD.

Besides impacting reimbursement, your MDS assessments determine your QMs. Your QMs are used for many purposes, including determining the QM domain star rating of your CMS star rating as well as guiding surveyors on what to take a closer look at during visits to your facility. To put it simply, the accuracy of your MDS assessments is extremely important.

Final Thoughts

MDS assessments are very time-sensitive. Not thoroughly completing and submitting them in a timely matter opens the door to potential tags and lost reimbursement. A high level of communication and coordination between the interdisciplinary team must occur to ensure not only the accuracy but the timeliness of the assessments.

There are several key meetings and systems that can be put in to place to ensure accuracy and proper reimbursement. A daily PPS meeting (soon to be PDPM meeting), a weekly Medicare or skilled meeting, a weekly case-mix meeting, and a monthly triple check meeting can all help protect revenue and ensure proper documentation, care, and reimbursement. There will be further discussion about these meetings in Chapter 25, but know now that administrators should take an active role in each of these meetings to ensure they are effective.

Though each state handles its reviews differently, at some point in time your MDSs will be scrutinized to ensure accuracy of payment. Monetary takebacks are common when inaccuracies and a lack of supporting documentation are found in the MDS assessments. Again, these reviews can result in significant revenue loss if a facility is not vigilant in ensuring that its documentation supports its claims in the MDS assessment. It is imperative that documentation always corroborates the information found in the MDS.

Finally, MDS assessments have been a growing area of examination during health inspections. Recently, in fact, an MDS-focused survey was created in which surveyors review MDS accuracy based on the care being provided.

Regardless of the survey type, inaccuracies found in the MDS can lead to tags and potential penalties and fines. At the end of the day, the goal of the facility should be to accurately document and capture all of the care being provided in order to enhance the quality of care, ensure accuracy of reimbursement, and protect the facility from risks.

KEY TAKEAWAYS

- Reimbursement systems can be very confusing and can take time to learn. Nevertheless, understanding the different payer types at your facility and the method they use to reimburse is important to your success as an administrator.
- An accurate and timely MDS assessment is important for many reasons, including proper reimbursement, QMs, quality care, and avoiding risks such as revenue takebacks, tags, and fines.
- MDS assessments are heavily scrutinized not only during health inspections but in other ways too, such as in verifying accuracy for proper reimbursement.

TASKS TO EXPAND YOUR LEARNING

- ☐ Help enter information on an MDS assessment for several residents.
- ☐ Conduct a BIMS, Pain Assessment, and PHQ-9 interview—all required on an MDS assessment.
- ☐ Ask the MDS nurse how they verify that CNA ADL documentation is accurate, and how often the facility trains on proper ADL documentation.
- ☐ Learn and study how Medicaid reimbursement works in your state. Explain what you learn to the department head team in a stand-up meeting.
- ☐ Review all of the facility's HMO contracts. Make a cheat sheet for each provider that lists the most important information in the contract, such as what

triggers different levels of payment as well as carve-outs (items you can bill additional money for, i.e. high-cost medications, special equipment, etc.)

COMMON POSITIONS IN THE DEPARTMENT

MDS coordinator (nurse) – This is an LVN/LPN/RN responsible for completing the MDS assessments. A good MDS nurse is excellent at meticulously combing through clinical records and finding the information needed to produce an accurate MDS assessment. They also should be great at documentation and should train other staff frequently on doing it properly. The MDS nurse often oversees and updates the clinical care plans for each resident, although at times this responsibility is given to ADONs or others. The MDS nurse must be organized and good at meeting deadlines, because MDS assessments must be completed on time to avoid penalties. Remember, late and/or incomplete assessments can result in the lowest reimbursement possible, regardless of care provided.

CHAPTER 20

Rehabilitation Services

Introduction

As a leader of a SNF, it is important to remember you don't sell products—you offer services. And to build a strong reputation and compete in the industry those services need to be top notch. One of the primary services you will provide is rehabilitation care.

Rehab is important to a SNF in many ways that will be discussed in this chapter. One big matter of importance that is sometimes overlooked: your facility's therapy services are at the crux of its reputation. Therapists spend much of their time working closely with short-term patients who return to the community. These patients interact with friends, families, physicians (during follow-up visits), and many other peers who may need the facility's services at some point. Without a doubt the experiences these short-term patients have at your facility will be shared with many in your community.

Often if short-term customers are thrilled with the therapy services they receive at your building, they will be happy with your facility in general even if something else went wrong during their stay. The opposite is also true. For this reason, your therapy department must strive to build a reputation of providing great care and getting people home quickly and safely.

Customer Satisfaction

For the most part, your customers should have nothing but good things to say about your rehab department. Though good therapists require hard work and effort from their patients, rehab is the place where customers can see progress, feel stronger and better about themselves, socialize and take their minds off their worries, and have a lot of fun. If you are getting more than an occasional random complaint about rehab at your facility, you should take a closer look at it quickly in order to fix the problem fast. Customer satisfaction scores regarding your therapy services should always rank at or near the top.

Skilled Services

Before we dive deeper into rehabilitation services, let's take a quick look at skilled services. Short-term care residents are often referred to as skilled patients. They are called "skilled" because in order to be covered by short term care insurance, such as Medicare or a Medicare replacement, they must have a skilled care need. Often this skilled care need is rehabilitation services. Per federal regulations, there are nine specific services that are defined as skilled services covered by Medicare for patients in a SNF. These include:

1. Intravenous or intramuscular injections and intravenous feeding
2. Enteral feeding (tube feeding) that comprises at least 26 percent of daily caloric intake and provides at least 501 milliliters of fluid per day
3. Nasopharyngeal and tracheostomy care
4. Insertion and sterile irrigation and replacement of suprapubic catheters
5. Application of dressings involving prescription medications and aseptic techniques
6. Treatment of extensive decubitus ulcers or other widespread skin disorder
7. Heat treatments which have been specifically ordered by a physician as part of an active treatment which requires observation by nurses to adequately evaluate the patient's progress

8. Initial phases of a regimen involving administration of medical gases
9. Rehabilitation nursing procedures, including the related teaching and adaptive aspects of nursing that are part of active treatment[1]

If a resident no longer has a need for skilled services, yet they are unsafe to transfer home or to a lower level of care, then typically they will transition to a long-term care resident within the SNF. If the SNF does not provide long-term care services, then they will find placement for this patient at a facility that does. Keep in mind that the insurance or payer source covering the short-term stay services will not cover the long-term stay services. Thus the resident will need alternate long-term care insurance such as Medicaid or another private insurance. Alternatively, the resident can pay out of pocket (private pay) for long-term care services.

Therapy for Short-Term Care Residents

As mentioned earlier, your therapist will spend much of their time with short-term (skilled) residents, as rehab plays a huge role in their recovery. Historically, rehabilitation services have also played an extremely significant role in reimbursement to the facility for short-term residents, but that will be changing drastically with the implementation of the PDPM reimbursement system. This new system will focus on the quality of therapy services more than on quantity. Regardless of the payment model, your therapy team members need to be

---

[1] See CMS Medicare Benefit Policy Manual, Pub. 100-02, Ch. 8, Sec. 30.3 https://www.cms.gov/Regulations-and-Guidance/Guidance/Manuals/Downloads/bp102c08.pdf and Ch. 7, Sec. 40.1 et seq. https://www.cms.gov/Regulations-and-Guidance/Guidance/Manuals/Downloads/bp102c07.pdf

organized, efficient, and wise in how they spend their time and deliver care in order to maximize the recovery of your patients.

It is important to keep in mind that short-term patients are typically covered by Medicare or a Medicare replacement plan. Coverage for skilled services with these plans normally allows an individual to have up to 100 days of care per spell of illness. This care is based on the needs and progress of the individual.

This doesn't mean 100 days of care is guaranteed; rather, it is the maximum amount that is covered. Short-term residents must meet certain skilled criteria during their entire stay in order to continue to be covered. As soon as they no longer meet the criteria—whether on day three of their stay or day 83, they should be discharged from skilled services.

Therapy teams should provide services that are reasonable and necessary for the recovery of their patients. SNFs are entrusted by those they care for to help them receive the best care their health insurance allows in the most efficient way possible. Helping to identify and remove barriers to progress in therapy (such as pain or drowsiness) is an important function of the interdisciplinary team. Again, the facility has an obligation to help each resident take full advantage of their limited benefits.

There are a few ways a therapist can deliver services. For example, they can provide individual one-on-one care, or they can provide therapy in a group setting (anywhere between two to four people at a time). There are different rules and regulations for how group therapy is captured and awarded between Medicare and the various HMO providers. Thus, it is important for the facility and rehab team to understand the differences and how group therapy will impact reimbursement to the facility. For some insurances it may be advantageous to provide group therapy while with others it may be prohibited.

Communication between the rehab and nursing depart-ments is vital when it comes to the care of short-term residents. Appointments, changes in medications, shower schedules, sleeping problems, pain, eating, and many other controllable factors can get in the way of a patient's ability to participate in therapy and receive great care. For this reason, nursing and rehab must be in constant communication so they can coordinate schedules to meet all the health care needs of the individual.

At the center of this communication is the relationship between the director of rehabilitation (DOR) and the DON. When these two key leaders work well together and communicate at a high level, others do the same. When there is friction and tension between these two leaders, it often trickles down. The administrator should keep an eye on this relationship and help it grow and strengthen as needed. When the nursing and rehab departments work well together, patients recover more quickly and are likely to have a great experience.

Therapy for Long-Term Care Residents

Rehab services should also play a big role in maintaining the health, quality of life, and independence of long-term residents. It can be common for therapists to get so focused on providing great care to the skilled population that they sometimes forget about the benefits of therapy to long-term care residents. Having certain systems and meetings in place to maintain a focus on the needs (including the therapy needs) of your long-term residents, is important and a great way to boost your overall quality of care.

A facility is most often reimbursed for therapy provided to long-term care residents through Medicare advantage plans or Medicare Part B. This reimbursement is based on the number of therapy units provided to a resident. Each therapy unit equals 15 minutes of therapy services. So, if a therapist provides 48 minutes of care, the facility could charge for three units. Under most circumstances, the number of therapy minutes provided to a long-term resident is lower than the number of minutes provided to a short-term patient during a given week. This is because the therapy needs for recovery and the therapy needs for maintenance are very different.

With current payment structures, profit margins for therapy given to long-term care residents are pretty low. However, therapy for long-term care residents with Medicaid can also play a substantial role in reimbursement levels in states that utilize a RUG system for reimbursement. As with short-term patients, the administrator must ensure that only the proper and appropriate therapy services are being provided to the long-term population.

Much like with short-term patients, communication between the nursing and rehab departments for long-term residents is paramount. When CNAs, nurses, or other staff notice a decline or increase in a resident's function and abilities, or if there are any changes in condition, the nursing team should have an easy way to share this information with the therapy team so they can evaluate and treat the resident as needed. SNFs are required to maintain the health and well-being of all their residents—failing to have a strong communication system between nursing and therapy will lead to poorer quality of care and missed opportunities to improve the quality of life for your long-term residents.

There are other common best practices to ensure that long-term residents are receiving proper attention and care from the therapy department. Some examples include scheduled quarterly therapy screens for each resident and providing a therapy screen each time a resident has a fall.

Therapy Financials

When looking at therapy financials, rather than using PPD for comparisons, many companies and skilled nursing leaders choose to use the per skilled day (PSD) metric for therapy number comparisons. So rather than dividing therapy numbers by the entire census at the facility, the numbers are divided only by the skilled census. This helps facilities make more accurate and reasonable comparisons.

There is no one perfect metric that adequately measures the overall performance of a therapy department, however there are a few meaningful therapy metrics administrators should pay close attention to. Productivity is one of those metrics, and it plays a key role in the performance of therapy at the facility. Therapy productivity is the amount of time a therapist spends treating patients in a day. Thus, assuming the facility is meeting all the documentation and other rules and regulations, the higher the productivity, the better.

Cost per minute is another common metric. It divides the costs of the department by the number of treatment minutes provided. Other common and useful metrics that indicate the performance of the therapy department include the therapy margin, long-term care caseload, and the average length of stay.

As with all departments in a SNF, managing the caseload and adjusting to census can be a challenge for the therapy department. Therapists are some of the most highly-compensated staff in the facility, so overtime in the therapy department is very costly. Having a strong PRN pool of therapists to meet the needs of patients (whether census is high or low) can help minimize overtime while always providing the appropriate amount of therapy care to those you serve.

Other Roles

Your therapy team can offer so much value to your facility beyond just providing therapy services to the residents. They can help train staff, improve the customer experience, educate families and the community on elderly care, build relationships and gain trust with local physicians, and really impact your facility's culture. Keep in mind that your therapy staff members have typically spent more time in school than any other professional group in the facility, so challenge them to extend their knowledge in order to make a positive impact.

Finally, the therapy department's role in meeting com-pliance rules and regulations is significant. With rules and regulations surrounding skilled stays and Medicare coverage as stringent as they are, the therapy department can and should do a lot to protect the facility against revenue takebacks and other compliance issues. The therapy team gathers and defines important information in the medical record that helps justify the services provided, including the prior level of function (PLOF), reasons why a skilled stay is needed, progress toward meeting certain goals, and discharge plans. All of these are key pieces of information that validate the provision of services to those within your care.

KEY TAKEAWAYS

- Therapy plays a significant role in the satisfaction of your short-term residents, who are often looking to recover quickly and return home. Most will share their experience at your facility with many others in the community who may soon need your services.
- Therapy departments should be focused on meeting both short-term and long-term patient needs.
- Excellent communication and teamwork between nursing and therapy is vital and starts with the relationship between the DOR and the DON.
- Key therapy metrics to measure the performance of your rehab team include productivity, cost per minute, therapy margin, long-term care caseload, and average length of stay. Monitoring these metrics and having goals to continually improve them will help elevate the therapy department's performance.

TASKS TO EXPAND YOUR LEARNING

- ☐ Learn about the different modalities used by each therapy discipline at your facility. Learn how each piece of equipment works in the therapy gym and how it benefits patients.
- ☐ Observe how the DOR manages and schedules therapy sessions and therapists' time, how they oversee the

plan and progress of each resident, and how they manage their own caseload.

☐ Determine what percentage of therapy provided by your team is individual, concurrent (one therapist to two patients), and group therapy (one therapist to three or more patients).

☐ Review the communication between the therapy and nursing departments, along with the screening practices of the therapy department. Determine if they are sufficient to meet long-term care needs or if improvement is needed.

☐ Look at the facility's average length of stay over the last few years and determine if it is increasing or decreasing. Talk to your team about why the length of stay matters to your health care partners, to the facility, and to those you take care of.

COMMON POSITIONS IN THE DEPARTMENT

Director of rehabilitation (DOR) – The DOR's primary responsibility is to oversee the therapy department, manage therapy staff, and ensure great rehab outcomes in areas such as productivity, efficiency, and customer satisfaction. DORs also participate in and contribute to important meetings, such as the daily PPS and triple check meetings. DORs do typically treat patients—the amount of time they spend doing this varies a lot between facilities. DORs can help with marketing and recruiting of physicians and can be big advocates for your facility's culture. A DOR can be licensed in any therapy discipline or can be a licensed therapy assistant. The right DOR can add a lot of value and contribute to a facility in a major way.

Physical therapist (PT) – A PT completes evaluations, develops therapy goals and plans, documents progress, completes therapy screenings, provides treatments, and oversees the work of physical therapy assistants. PTs focus on gross motor movements such as standing, walking, and lifting.

Physical therapy assistant (PTA) – A PTA's main responsibility is to provide treatments and care to patients. Their work is overseen by a PT and they follow the plan of care outlined. PTAs are more hands-on in their work and don't have as many paperwork obligations and responsibilities as a PT.

Occupational therapist (OT or OTR) – An OT completes evaluations, develops therapy goals and plans, documents progress, completes therapy screenings, provides treatments, and oversees the work of occupational therapy assistants. OTs focus on helping and improving self-help skills and ADLs such as dressing, feeding, and toileting.

Certified occupational therapy assistant (COTA) – An occupational therapy assistant's main responsibility is to provide treatments and care for patients. Their work is overseen by an OT, and they follow the plan of care outlined. COTAs provide more hands-on work and don't have as many paperwork obligations and responsibilities as a OT.

Speech language pathologist (speech therapist) – A speech language pathologist or speech therapist completes evaluations, develops therapy goals and plans, documents progress, conducts therapy screenings, and provides treatments. They focus on acquisition and use of language, cognition, and swallowing.

Therapy tech – A therapy tech assists the entire department as well as individual therapists with tasks assigned. This may include preparing residents for treatment, making phone calls, doing data entry, assisting with treatments, and keeping the therapy equipment clean and in good working order. Therapy techs try to do all they can to lighten the load of others in the

therapy department so they can stay productive. The use of
therapy techs varies between facilities; many facilities do not
have any, while others may have a few.

CHAPTER 21

Business Office and Accounts Receivable

Introduction

It's one thing to provide care and services and then book revenue for those services each month, but it's a whole other issue to actually collect the money. Uncollected revenue and poor business office results can ruin the stellar performance in other aspects of the facility. As an administrator, you can make certain your business office won't bring you down by taking an active role in collections at your facility and by hiring the right business office manager (BOM).

Business Office Definitions

To begin, let's define a few common business office terms and important metrics.

Bad debt can be a little different for each organization, but essentially it is an expense based on revenues that are presumed uncollectable. A high bad debt expense due to poor collection efforts can ruin an otherwise strong financial month.

DSO, or days sales outstanding, is the amount of time it takes the facility to collect cash. The lower the better: this means the facility is getting cash in its hands quicker.

Aging is the amount of time a revenue item has been on the books. If a facility provided services to a resident six months ago and hasn't collected the cash, the aging on that revenue would be around 180 days. The cleaner the aging, meaning the quicker a facility is collecting money and fixing any booking errors, the better.

Cash collection percentage is the amount of cash collected during the month divided by the revenue booked the previous month. Under normal circumstances, a cash collections percentage of 100% or slightly higher is a common goal for many facilities.

Bad debt as a percentage of revenue is a very common metric facilities look at to gauge business office performance. This number is derived by taking the bad debt expense for the month (or quarter, year, etc.) and dividing it by the total revenue for the month (or quarter or year). A common goal is to be below 1%.

All the metrics listed above are correlated and impact each other in one way or another. Many are lagging indicators which means they don't represent present-day performance, but rather reflect what performance had been in the past. The one number that will eventually drive success in all of them is the percentage of cash collections. Thus, staying on top of cash collections throughout the month is a must for BOMs and administrators.

Good Cash Collections

Good cash collections start with a consistent and effective weekly accounts receivable (AR) review. This review typically involves the administrator and the BOM. Together they review important accounts, such as those with the highest dollars owed to the facility. They also plan next steps to collect on those accounts.

Two important tasks for the administrator during this meeting are taking good notes and following up on commitments made during the previous review. When a facility is struggling, the administrator may decide to do AR reviews more frequently. A consistent and thorough AR review will help the facility make progress on difficult accounts and improve overall cash collections.

Another important way to ensure good cash collections is to accurately bill insurances *the first time*. This is sometimes referred to as *clean billing* and often requires a BOM to slow down and take a little extra time to ensure all "t's" are crossed and "i's" are dotted. But it is well worth the effort. Part of this process includes meticulously keeping an accurate census so proper days are invoiced.

Each payer requires different information in order to properly bill them. Understanding how the different payer types need to be billed and then submitting invoices correctly and efficiently will ensure the cash flows in.

Frequent follow-up is another very important route to good cash collections. When a bill isn't being paid, the BOM needs to find out why. When someone doesn't have an answer to a question about payment to the facility, the BOM must stay persistent until they are provided answers. Staying organized and routinely following up on uncollected accounts will lead to greater success.

One final way to facilitate good cash collections is ensuring the BOM takes an active role in important meetings. To bill many insurances, such as Medicare, a facility must meet all the rules and regulations regarding the necessary documentation to bill. Certain necessary items such as qualifying stay dates, ARDs, and Medicare certifications are examples of documentation that should be discussed and verified during daily PPS meetings and monthly triple check meetings. A BOM is the backstop to ensure everything is in place for proper billing.

Two Common Mistakes

One very common mistake that can lead to poor cash collections and poor business office results is failing to verify insurance and/or obtain a prior authorization for coverage before admitting patients. Sometimes in the haste to meet the needs of patients and referral sources, a facility admits haphazardly. In other words, they admit without verifying benefits.

When appropriate systems are in place and people are trained properly, the verification of benefits or requests for prior authorizations shouldn't take long or be too arduous of a process. However, failing to verify insurance or receive proper authorization can lead to a non-paying admission and a lot of business office headaches.

A second common mistake is accepting a high number of Medicaid-pending patients *without* having a system in place to track and follow through with enrollment. Let me emphasize that the issue isn't in accepting the Medicaid-pending patient (for many facilities it is a good intelligent risk and a possible niche to actively accept them). The problem is when there isn't an effective system in place to see the Medicaid application process through to the end.

Someone in the facility must be assigned to take responsibility for Medicaid-pending resident applications and continuously follow up until Medicaid is approved. This person could be someone in the business office, but at a minimum the BOM should work closely with them to ensure successful follow-through and completion of the process.

Business Office Tidbits

BOMs can also play an important role in customer service. Most people don't like to be billed or have to pay out money. Good BOMs are persistent for sure—this is a must—but they are persistent in a way that is confident and professional. Good BOMs are excellent at responding with patience and concern to angry, confused, rude, or less-than-happy customers who don't really want to deal with money matters (which is most of them). However, BOMs must also stay consistent and honest about collection efforts.

In regards to DSO, the speed by which different payers pay varies a lot. For this reason, DSO standards among facilities can vary a great deal. Facilities with a high number of HMO patients will collect much slower and therefore have a much higher DSO than facilities with a lot of private pay patients who consistently pay at the beginning of each month, for example. The key to DSO success is accurate and timely billing.

In terms of regulatory compliance and the business office, facilities are required to offer and establish a trust fund account for each resident. This is in essence a bank account that the facility manages for the resident. A resident trust fund audit is conducted each year by the state to verify that all rules and regulations pertaining to the resident trust fund are being followed. Some common issues that arise during these audits include a lack of proper receipts for expenditures and a lack of timely refunds.

KEY TAKEAWAYS

- Collections are very important to the success of a facility!
- Good cash collections start with a consistent and effective weekly AR Review.
- Business office performance is normally measured by important key metrics such as bad debt as a percentage of revenue, DSO, and cash collections.
- Some common culprits for poor business office performance include a lack of monitoring by the administrator, a lack of billing accuracy and timeliness, admitting patients without verifying benefits, a lack of follow-through with Medicaid applications, and a failure to continuously follow up on accounts.

TASKS TO EXPAND YOUR LEARNING

- ☐ Participate in all billing efforts for all payer sources, including making collection calls, updating the cash log, preparing and sending proper invoices, following up on accounts, verifying benefits, answering invoice questions, etc.
- ☐ Run the common working file for multiple residents (a common working file is a tool used by CMS to maintain records for individual beneficiaries enrolled. The system is used by SNFs to determine eligibility and usage of

benefits). Learn to understand the information found in the common working file.

- [ ] Review the aging of the facility's revenue. List the different payer types and identify those that appear to be the most problematic for the facility. Try to identify the reasons why they are the most challenging and brainstorm ideas for improvement with the business office team.
- [ ] Review the findings from the facility's last trust fund audit and ensure that deficiencies have been corrected.
- [ ] Review the process for tracking census and making sure it is accurate.
- [ ] Learn how bad debt works at your facility and how the bad debt expense is determined each month.
- [ ] Hold weekly AR reviews with your BOM.

COMMON POSITIONS IN THE DEPARTMENT

Business office manager (BOM) – Leads and oversees all collection efforts in the facility, including helping to ensure proper documentation is in place to bill. Spends time attending and participating in important meetings such as PPS and triple check meetings. Prepares and sends accurate and timely invoices; makes collection calls; explains billing, benefits, and invoices; manages journal entries, write-offs, adjustments, etc. Investigates and corrects unpaid or rejected invoices. Manages other business office team members. The BOM is a key leader who has a significant impact on the facility's success.

Assistant business office manager (ABOM) – Helps the BOM fulfill their responsibilities and takes on tasks as assigned by the BOM. May be assigned to manage and oversee collection efforts for certain payer sources. Not all facilities have an ABOM.

CHAPTER 22

Financial Management

Introduction

As the administrator of a SNF, one of your primary responsibilities is to ensure the financial success of your facility. Unstable and inconsistent financial performance often leads to a high level of uncertainty and instability in *every* aspect of the building. Understand that poor financial performance puts the residents, staff, and everyone who relies on the facility at risk.

There are many ways to ensure financial success, including building the facility's reputation for great clinical care, cultivating a strong culture that helps you attract and retain the right team members, and having great survey and compliance results. These are all important and go hand in hand with closely managing and monitoring facility spending and reimbursement. In this chapter, we will take a close look at simple things you can do to run a financially-successful facility.

Two Approaches to Financials

Too frequently, administrators fail because they don't take the responsibility of financial success seriously enough. They may prioritize other things first. In these instances, it important to remember the words of Sister Irene Krause when she proclaimed, "no margin no mission." It is hard to provide great care when the facility is struggling to keep the lights on for example. At the end of the day, an administrator must ensure the financial viability of the operation in order to be able to meet the needs of all those who have placed their trust in the facility.

For every administrator that doesn't properly prioritize financial performance, however, there is another who will do the exact opposite and *only* show interest in the facility's financials. Both approaches are a mistake, and both lead to too many administrators' eventual downfall.

Administrators with the tendency to exclusively focus on financial performance need to understand that there may be many individuals within their facility who are not all that interested in financial information, or even financial success. They must recognize that most caregivers go into health care because they want to help those in need and not because they want to make money.

This does not mean that financial information should not be shared with the team, or that it should never be spoken about. In fact, just the opposite is true. Many department heads and other staff will do a lot to help improve the financial well-being of a facility once they know how. Administrators who ignore financial performance or fail to guide their staff to greater fiscal control and responsibility hurt their team's ability to make improvements and work smarter.

The point of all of this is that messages *only* about money won't resonate with or inspire the majority of your staff, but neither will messages completely devoid of fiscal results and stewardship. Sending either of these types of messages will prevent you from rallying and engaging your teams. For this reason, a wise administrator speaks frequently to their staff about their opportunity to serve and help others in need while also connecting the dots between financial success and the facility's ability to provide the highest level of quality care. The two are inseparable, and the administrator must help everyone understand this fact.

With that out of the way, let's look at some basic financial principles that are critical to your success.

PPD and PSD

The most common metric used in the SNF industry is PPD, which, as discussed in Chapter 1, means "per patient day." Using this metric allows very different facilities to compare apples to apples. PPD is looked at most commonly in two ways:

1) Dollars PPD—how many dollars you spend on something per patient per day.

2) Hours PPD—how many hours you use per patient per day.

Calculating PPD is simple: take the total dollar amount or total hours used and divide it by the total number of patient days. For example, if I had 3,000 patient days in the month of November and spent $15,000 on food during the month, I'd take the $15,000 and divide it by 3,000 patient days. The result: $5 PPD on food.

As another example, let's say that my dietary staff worked 1,200 hours in November. To calculate the hours PPD for dietary, I'd divide the 1,200 hours by the number of patient days (3,000), which would give me 0.4 hours PPD.

A PPD measurement is important because it essentially removes all the variables that exist between facilities and allows for meaningful comparisons. In some cases, the PSD (per skilled day) metric may also be used to provide more meaningful comparisons for a particular cost category. Since PSD refers to *skilled* days, it removes the long-term patients from the calculation, thus isolating the total number of skilled days.

For example, let's say in the month of April you average 25 skilled patients a day for a total of 750 (25 x 30 days) skilled days for the month. Now let's say the facility spent $75,000 in therapy wages in April. If you take this dollar amount and divide it by the total number of skilled days for the month, your therapy wages would be $100 PSD. Some common cost categories that may be looked at on a PSD basis include therapy, pharmacy, and lab.

Trends in PPDs and PSDs are almost always closely scrutinized to determine if a facility is improving or declining. An administrator may believe they are doing really well with supply purchases because they've cut spending by $2,000 from one month to another, but others might disagree when they notice that expenses per patient day actually increased due to a census decline. What this means for you as an administrator is that you can't focus on whole dollars only—you need to think more about costs and hours in relation to census. It only makes sense for whole dollars to go down when the facility is taking care of fewer patients.

The challenge for an administrator is to find ways not only to decrease overall costs but also to make spending go down on a per patient day basis. This requires frequent monitoring and adjusting based on census levels at the facility.

Cost Control and Spend Down System

As we learned in Chapter 19, there are two ways to improve your bottom line (or net income). You can increase your revenue and/or decrease your expenditures. Since we've discussed PPDs, let's now start with cost control and then we will move to revenue growth.

The most significant expenditure in any facility is staff wages. Typically, wages make up at least 65% of total dollars spent at a SNF. For this reason, a *daily* labor review is extremely critical. As mentioned in Chapter 11, effective daily labor reviews consist of: 1) monitoring appropriate clocking in and out at the beginning and end of shifts, 2) monitoring proper clocking in and out for lunch breaks, and 3) monitoring and minimizing overtime. Let me reiterate that staffing appropriately is the number-one way to control costs and reduce spending.

After wages, other significant spending categories include pharmacy, patient supplies, and food/supplements spending. Monitoring and controlling spending on these expenditures alone will go a long way in improving your facility's financial performance. When it comes to reducing spending, these cost categories, along with wages, are good places to start. Don't get hung up on saving a penny here or there on housekeeping supplies for example when your pharmacy spending is out of control. Too many administrators try to put out a small flame when a huge fire is roaring behind them. Focus on the big stuff first and then move to the fine-tuning.

Providing clear budgets to department leaders and tracking spending through a spend-down system will greatly enhance your ability to monitor and control costs. A spend-down system works like a checkbook: the department leader is given a budget at the beginning of the month and tracks spending by subtracting each expenditure from the total budget. This system allows the department head to see how much money they have left for the month at any given time and challenges them to stay within budget.

Asking department heads to hand in an updated copy of their monthly spend-down each week makes it easy for an administrator to keep an eye on costs and be proactive in helping department heads meet their budgets.

Other ways to control costs include eliminating waste (i.e. misuse of supplies, theft, food waste) and reviewing vendor contracts. Having systems to help you with both of these can really reduce your spending.

Remember that in the skilled nursing industry, margins are tight and every penny counts. This does not mean an administrator must be a penny pincher. A facility must spend money to make money. However, careful consideration should be made about expenditures because there is only so much money to go around, and dollars spent add up quickly. Too many facilities struggle and fail to provide great care because of out-of-control, undisciplined spending.

Revenue Growth

There are many factors to look at when considering how to increase revenue. Census growth is perhaps the most common and seemingly easiest way to increase your revenue, and it's a great place to start. In general, the more customers you serve, the higher your revenue will be. However, administrators must keep in mind that increasing the facility's census isn't the only way to grow revenue.

Reimbursement amounts are another very important factor to consider. Remember that not all admissions are created equal, as some payer sources generate a lot more daily revenue than others. Let's say my Medicaid revenue per patient day is $150 and my Medicare revenue per patient day is $550. If my total census increases by 10 patients in comparison to last month, however my Medicaid census grew by 15 and my skilled census dropped by five, then my total revenue will have decreased even though my census went up.

Often facilities increase their census but only grow their revenue by an insignificant amount because reimbursement rates decrease. Too many administrators are surprised to see their monthly financial performance is poor after an increase in census.

Let's take a look at another example of this. Imagine your facility averages 100 patients a day with an average payment of $200 a day in July. Then, in August, your census explodes and you average 110 patients a day, but reimbursement drops to $180 because you don't do as good of a job capturing the services provided to the residents. Which month will have higher revenue?

In this simple example, your facility will have higher revenue during the month with the lower census!

In addition to a dip in reimbursement rate, often what happens when census goes up is facility staff begin to spend more, assuming there is more money to go around. What people fail to realize is an increase in census does not guarantee an increase in revenue. As you can imagine, this behavior and lack of fiscal understanding and discipline leads to poor financial performance.

Hopefully you see the importance of reimbursement rates to your revenue. Doing all you can to receive proper reimbursement by taking credit for all of the services your facility is providing is paramount to financial success.

Reviewing for proper reimbursement happens during important meetings such as the daily PPS, weekly case-mix, and monthly triple check meetings. Too often, administrators and facilities don't take these meetings seriously enough and thus fail to take credit for the work they do—resulting in lower reimbursement and less revenue.

Medicare Part B is another revenue source to consider. Part B revenue is most often secured by providing therapy services to long-term care patients. However, it can also come from billing for other services provided to long-term residents, such as vaccinations and wound care supplies, for example.

Carve-outs from HMO contracts—where additional items and services can be billed and reimbursed per your facility contracts—are another potential revenue opportunity. Understanding the carve-outs for each contract and how to bill them is a must.

The average length of stay in the facility can also have huge ramifications for revenue. Focusing on eliminating unnecessary re-hospitalizations and providing great customer service upon admission (so that patients stay and receive appropriate care) can improve this metric significantly and bolster revenue.

There are also other alternative and creative ways to increase revenue, including renting out space in the facility, selling meals or facility merchandise, and owning vending machines at the facility, just to name a few.

Final Tidbits

Another important practice for administrators is scrubbing and reviewing profit and loss (P&L) statements each month. This practice will not only allow you to catch any accounting mistakes, but it will also help you understand your facility better and identify opportunities for improvement. This detailed monthly review of the facility financial documents is a must.

Frequent financial comparisons are also extremely helpful in finding trends and areas to focus on and improve. If you belong to a larger corporation, ask to review comparisons between your facility's PPDs and other sister facilities' PPDs. Also, frequently compare your facility's past and current financials. How did this May's performance compare to last May's? How about this month versus last month or this quarter versus the previous quarters? Are PPDs improving or getting worse, and why? It can be difficult to recognize the areas where you are improving, or the areas where you need to improve, without performing frequent comparisons and reviews.

Remember, no other leader is primarily as responsible for the facility's financial success as you are. Sure, every leader plays a part, and can and should be striving for good financial outcomes. But it is up to you as the administrator to ensure that your facility's leaders understand their role in impacting financial performance. Good administrators are often deep in the details of their financials and know where action must be taken to improve.

KEY TAKEAWAYS

- Ensuring the financial viability of the facility is a primary role of an administrator.
- Both ignoring or talking exclusively about financials will make it difficult for an administrator to rally their team.
- PPD is the most common financial metric used in the industry because it strips out all external factors and allows very different facilities or very different points in time at a facility to be compared.
- Wages are the biggest expense in a facility followed by pharmacy, patient supplies, and food/supplements spending. Controlling these cost areas will yield big results in financial performance.
- A spend down system is a good way for administrators to monitor spending.
- Census growth and reimbursement rates will have the greatest impact on the facility's revenue.
- Margins are tight in health care, especially in skilled nursing. For this reason, financials must be monitored closely by the administrator.

TASKS TO EXPAND YOUR LEARNING

- ☐ Review and become extremely familiar with the financial statements, reports, and documents of the facility. Go through each financial document line-by-line and make sure you understand what each line means.

☐ Scrub your most recent financial statement by looking at every expense and revenue category line-by-line. Ensure that the financial statement is accurate.

☐ Make a spreadsheet that compares PPD trends for the facility over the last four quarters and over the last 12 months in each major cost and revenue category. What trends stand out?

☐ Review established budgets. Make a list of budgets that are and are not being met consistently. Then review the facility spend-down system and improve it if necessary.

COMMON POSITIONS IN THE DEPARTMENT

Administrator – Oversees all aspects of a SNF and is responsible for all outcomes, including clinical, culture, compliance and regulatory, and financial results. Has a primary responsibility of ensuring the financial viability of the operation. Ensures that the facility is always adhering to all rules and regulations and is doing business in an ethical way. Is responsible for the safety and well-being of all residents, staff, and anyone who enters the facility's doors.

CHAPTER 23

Accounts Payable

Introduction

Accounts payable (AP) is an important system in a SNF. How you review and pay bills can help you save thousands of dollars. Though most vendors are not trying to be fraudulent or pull a fast one on you, it is important to remember that many companies are not in business to produce accurate invoices. Mistakes happen with invoicing (SNFs do it all the time, too) and for this reason alone it is important to review all of your invoices before paying them.

Unfortunately, there are some dishonest people and companies out there. It is not unheard of for an unethical business to send facilities products that no one ever ordered and then try to charge for them. Or they might not even send any products at all, but still send a bill.

Facilities that simply pay all invoices without close review can end up paying for inaccurate or untrue invoicing.

AP Processing

Your AP processor plays an important role in your facility by ensuring the accuracy and validity of invoices. Often this important task is handled by the HR/payroll director, ABOM, or even the receptionist. Whoever it is, the AP processor must be well-organized and attentive in reviewing invoices to verify accuracy. They must also be willing to work closely with the administrator and others in order to carefully comb over all invoices.

There are a wide variety of systems that can be put into place to ensure accuracy and to review invoices, but here is a common and effective one:

1. All invoices go first to the AP processor. They review the invoice for accuracy, including checking the date of invoice, date of services, services or product provided, and whether the vendor is known or recognized.
2. Next, the AP processor gives each department head a batch of the invoices pertaining to their department and budget for approval. For example, all the food invoices would go to the dietary supervisor for review and approval. The department head reviews each invoice for accuracy and validity and initials the invoice and returns it to the AP processor.
3. The AP processor then puts together a weekly batch of all the invoices received during the week (and reviewed by the department heads) and reviews them with the administrator.
4. The administrator signs off on each approved invoice and identifies invoices that need further investigation.
5. The AP processor submits the approved invoices for payment and investigates the others.

Though rarely the highlight of an administrator's day, reviewing invoices is an important responsibility. Administrators who don't review their invoices consistently will spend thousands of unnecessary dollars a month.

A best practice is to set aside time to review a batch of invoices each week. This way the task remains manageable and is easier to stay on top of.

KEY TAKEAWAYS

- Failing to review and scrutinize all invoices before payment can cost the facility thousands of dollars.
- A good AP system is one that requires invoices to be reviewed by several different leaders before payment including the department head who made the purchase and the administrator.
- Administrators should review invoices weekly and must check for accuracy and validity.

TASKS TO EXPAND YOUR LEARNING

- ☐ Create an AP batch on your own and handle a bill all the way through the process, from receipt to payment.
- ☐ Create a spreadsheet of vendors that includes how often the vendor invoices the facility (i.e. weekly, semimonthly, monthly, quarterly) and the terms of payment (how quickly the facility needs to pay the invoice, i.e. within 14 days, 30 days, 60 days). Next, add in the dollar amount paid to each vendor for the last three months and sort the list from the most dollars spent to the least.

COMMON POSITIONS IN THE DEPARTMENT

Accounts payable (AP) processor – This designation is usually given to an existing leader in the facility, such as the HR/payroll director, ABOM, or even the receptionist. This person is responsible for handling all vendor invoices and submission of payment. The AP processor helps oversee and improve the facility's AP systems. They handle vendor questions and concerns about payment and set new vendors up to be paid. They work closely with the administrator and follow systems to verify the accuracy of invoices. They follow up with vendors about questions, requests for corrections, or deletions of invoices.

CHAPTER 24

Central Supply, Equipment, and Staffing

Introduction
In this chapter we will cover three different topics that can cost the facility a lot of money if not managed well by an organized leader. And though these three areas are pretty different from one another, it isn't unusual for one person to be in charge of all of them. Nonetheless, each facility is unique, and these responsibilities may also be divided up between different leaders. Let's go ahead and dive into each.

Supplies
As an administrator, supplies can cause you problems in two big ways. First, not having sufficient supplies can lead to poor care and disgruntled staff. The leader you place in charge of supplies must be good at managing them, including ordering effectively, stocking supply closets frequently, and taking inventory regularly. No matter the reason, not having supplies on hand erodes the trust and confidence families, patients, and staff have in your facility. You must make it your goal to always have the supplies your team needs to take great care of your residents.

The second problem is that supplies can potentially cost you a lot—so there must be systems in place to manage spending. Having a budget and a spend-down for your supplies is vital. As an administrator, it is a good idea to have the person in charge of supplies give you weekly spending updates so that you can oversee how they are doing in meeting their monthly budget. A simple way to do this is by requiring a copy of their updated spend-down each week. Getting weekly updates will help you be proactive in helping your leader manage costs and meet budget.

Supply Spending

There are several reasons why supply spending might be high. Let's take a look at some of them.

One thing to consider when spending is high in a facility is the acuity of the residents receiving care. For example, if you have a lot of residents with wounds, this may cause your supply expenses to be higher than normal because wound care products tend to be expensive. High spending on supplies strictly due to high acuity is an acceptable problem to have because the reimbursement and additional revenue received will nearly always make up for the higher costs of supplies.

Another cause of high spending may be waste. For example, staff could be grabbing the wrong size gloves and throwing them in the trash before grabbing the right ones, or they could be throwing dirty linen in the trash rather than the hamper. Supplies may also be falling on the floor, making them unsanitary to use and thus getting thrown away. Look for opportunities to minimize waste when expenses are high.

Improper supply use is another common occurrence that increases costs. For example, maybe a CNA is putting a large-size brief on every patient regardless of their need for a smaller size. Since larger briefs cost more, you will be wasting money on patients who need a small- or medium-size brief. This can drive costs up.

Hoarding supplies is also common in many facilities. This most often occurs when staff feel there may not be enough supplies, so they keep extras on hand by hiding them at the top of resident closets or in the back of drawers just in case supplies run out. This leads to a surplus of supplies throughout the facility and a lot of waste.

Standing orders can be another cause of high costs. One facility I worked with had a standing order of supplies that was shipped to them each week. When diving into why their costs were so high we discovered a large room in the back full of surplus supplies. The building was literally spending thousands of unnecessary dollars each month on supplies they already had in abundance!

Finally, theft is a possible reason for increased spending. Supplies can be expensive and sometimes staff or families take them home for personal use. Monitoring for and eliminating theft can help you control spending on supplies.

When supply spending seems high, take a close look at each of these common causes and then make adjustments and offer training as necessary.

Supply Distribution and Contracts

Although it may seem simple enough, how supplies are distributed in a facility can lead to both of the big problems described above (running out of supplies and spending too much on supplies). Plenty of facilities struggle with and/or simply ignore the significance of the supply distribution system. This system is critical because it impacts nearly everyone in the facility. Making sure supplies are available and always accessible to staff while also preventing misuse and/or theft can be a real challenge. Thus, taking the time to determine and evaluate what works best for your facility is time well spent. And frequently tweaking and adjusting the distribution process with your central supply leader and caregivers in order to improve the system is a good idea.

One final consideration about supplies is that some facilities use a PPD purchasing system, and others use a fee-for-service system. A PPD contract for supplies means a company essentially provides all the basic supplies needed for your patients at a predetermined price per patient per day. The advantage of this is that when census is down, supply costs theoretically go down too. A PPD contract also makes costs more predictable and can save the central supply leader time. One drawback of this type of contract is that supplies are often needed outside of the PPD formulary, which can negatively impact the potential positives of such an arrangement.

The advantages of a fee-for-service-system (paying for supplies as needed) are that it allows you to shop around for the best pricing and it gives you control over who you purchase from and what products you order. The drawback is that your central supply leader needs to be more on top of things. They will need to spend time monitoring pricing, controlling inventory levels, weighing different options, and using their budget wisely.

Equipment

Now let's talk equipment. Equipment can add up and can also cost a facility a lot of money. Sometimes the oversight of equipment is not specifically assigned to one person in a facility and so there may be very little accountability or ownership of it. As the administrator, make sure it is clear whose duty and responsibility it is to order, return, keep up with, and maintain equipment.

Having a good equipment tracking system in place is critical. When renting equipment, the facility should know the cost of the rental as well as how to return the equipment. The person assigned to the oversight of the equipment should frequently check on patients with rental equipment to make sure it is still needed, and they must return the equipment as quickly as possible. Many facilities spend thousands of dollars on rental equipment that sits in closets unused. Other times rental equipment goes missing, causing the facility to have to pay for it. Keeping a close eye on rental equipment is very important.

Negotiating pricing on rental equipment is also a good idea. There is often a significant difference in the cost of equipment between companies. Just because a company has the best pricing for one piece of equipment, it doesn't mean they will have the best pricing for all other equipment. Taking the time to find the best deal for each piece of equipment is usually worth the effort.

Rental equipment companies are often smaller local businesses whose main purpose is to provide health care equipment to facilities such as yours. Sometimes these companies do not always have the best tracking and billing systems in place and their invoices may have errors. One facility I worked at was charged eight additional months for a piece of equipment that had been returned! However, since invoices weren't monitored closely and equipment wasn't tracked well, the facility continued to pay for it. This is another reason why tracking closely on your end is a good idea to ensure you are charged appropriately for rented equipment.

Maintaining a list of equipment owned by the facility and conducting routine maintenance to keep the equipment in good working order is important. Too many oxygen concentrators burn up simply because filters are not cleaned and changed when needed. And too many pieces of equipment are rented when the facility owns that exact piece of equipment—it just happens to be hiding in a closet, or staff isn't aware the facility owns it.

Finally, equipment cleaning can also be a problem for many facilities. Often housekeepers may be scared to touch equipment for fear of damaging it, accidentally turning it off, or causing harm to the patient. For me it was always easiest to have housekeepers trained on how to clean equipment and make this part of their daily routine and responsibilities. However, some facilities shift this responsibility to CNAs or even nurses who are more comfortable around the equipment. The most important thing is that this task is assigned to someone and it is taken care of so dirty equipment does not jeopardize care.

Staffing

Now, let's talk staffing. There are many different ways to staff a building. Some facilities follow a four days on, two days off schedule, while others do Monday through Friday schedules with different staff on the weekends. Some do two 12-hour shifts each day while others do three 8-hours shifts. Some have their first shift start as early as 5 a.m. or as late as 9 a.m. There is no one-size-fits-all or the best way to staff every building.

Finding the staffing method that works best for your facility, the local community, and your entire team is important. There is a lot to take into consideration when deciding how to schedule staff. Work closely with your best team members, including staff who work the floor, when making scheduling decisions. Keep in mind that a schedule that will help you attract and retain the best talent should nearly always be the number-one priority when deciding how to best schedule your team.

Your facility's staffing coordinator will play a key role in a few ways. First, how they treat staff, communicate with them, motivate them, trust them, and work with them will help shape your culture and the overall experience your staff have at the facility. Second, the impact the staffing coordinator has on your dollars spent on wages at the facility is huge. The staffing coordinator must always ensure that the facility is appropriately staffed while working to control overtime usage and/or overstaffing.

A good staffing coordinator can be an invaluable team member at your facility and should be made to feel like an important part of the team.

Finally, don't forget to find ways to give your staffing coordinator breaks from time to time. This is a position that tends to burn out quickly, so keep a watchful eye on them and take good care of them.

KEY TAKEAWAYS

- Not having adequate supplies or running short even once can hurt your facility's reputation.
- Supply costs add up quickly, so you must have good systems in place to control, distribute, and monitor them.
- Without a good tracking system, a lot of money can be wasted on equipment.
- The staffing coordinator plays a key role in your facility and impacts not only dollars spent on wages but also the overall experience of your team.

TASKS TO EXPAND YOUR LEARNING

- ☐ Work as the staffing coordinator for a day. Carry the on-call phone, make adjustments to the schedule as needed, post the daily staffing, check and maintain sign in/out sheets, report on daily hours, and review detailed labor hour reports and overtime reports.
- ☐ Review the staffing schedules. Is there any overtime built into the schedules (meaning someone is scheduled over 40 hours a week [or over 8 hours a day in some states] before the schedule even begins)?
- ☐ Create the next schedule for the nursing staff.
- ☐ Order, stock, and distribute supplies for a day. Conduct a supply inventory and check par levels.

- ☐ Identify a few nursing supply vendors and compare pricing. Negotiate better pricing than what the facility currently has.
- ☐ Look in closets, dresser drawers, and clean/dirty utility cabinets for hoarding of supplies.
- ☐ Order and track all rental equipment for a week.
- ☐ Identify a few equipment companies and compare pricing on the equipment most used by the facility. Negotiate better pricing for equipment rentals.
- ☐ Update the equipment inventory list by "putting eyes" on all pieces of equipment and checking to ensure they are all in good working order.

COMMON POSITIONS IN THE DEPARTMENT

Central supply director – Holds the primary responsibility for supplies, including ordering and maintaining adequate supplies, stocking and distributing supplies, completing inventory and maintaining par levels, negotiating and finding the best pricing for supplies, and adhering to a supplies budget. As a reminder, these responsibilities are often given to other leaders in the facility such as ADONs or the staffing coordinator.

Equipment director – Responsibilities include ordering, tracking, and maintaining the facility equipment, negotiating and finding the best pricing for equipment, returning rental equipment as soon as possible, and meeting equipment budgets. These responsibilities are often given to other leaders in the facility such as ADONs, maintenance and/or housekeeping directors, central supply directors, or the staffing coordinator.

Staffing coordinator – Responsibilities include creating and communicating nursing staff schedules, setting up interviews and screening potential candidates for open positions, finding coverage for all shifts to ensure consistency in care, helping train CNAs and assisting them in their duties, working the floor when shorthanded, reporting on daily staffing numbers, and tracking hours to minimize overtime and meet budgeted hours. The staffing coordinator often has additional duties such as overseeing central supplies and equipment, picking up shifts on the floor, or other responsibilities as assigned. A staffing coordinator is often a CNA or LVN. Staffing can also be handled by the DON, DSD, ADONs, or other nursing administration team members.

CHAPTER 25

Crucial Meetings

Introduction

Many people dread meetings. What I've learned is that most team members in a SNF follow their leader's example in terms of his or her attitude toward meetings. If the leader's attitude about a meeting is upbeat and positive, the attitudes of others toward the meeting will be similar.

I've also observed that one of the best ways to improve a meeting is for an administrator to simply attend and participate.

Crucial SNF meetings can be mundane and repetitive, however when done effectively they can be a powerful force in helping the administrator run a successful facility. Therefore, your good attitude toward meetings and your attendance at them is vital.

Holding Effective Meetings

When it comes to making meetings effective and impactful, there are three key things to remember.

First, the purpose of the meeting must be clear to all. If people don't know why a meeting is being held, it can become easier for them to disengage and not make the meeting a priority. When the purpose of the meeting isn't clear it is also easier for people to get distracted and go off on tangents that don't contribute to the meeting.

Second, people must understand their specific role in the meeting. Many meetings are ineffective because people do not understand their role in moving the meeting along and working toward its overall objective. Too often in SNF meetings, different leaders end up duplicating their efforts—thus making the meeting longer than it needs to be and less effective than it ought to be. For example, during a daily PPS meeting, only one person needs to verify the qualifying stay dates while others look at other important information they've been assigned to. If everyone is digging up the qualifying stay dates and then everyone turns to the ADL documentation, then everyone looks at the therapy minutes, your meeting will be a lot longer than it needs to be and it will waste a lot of time. Instead, clearly define assignments in terms of who should be looking for what in the clinical record. This will allow meetings to run much more efficiently.

Third, avoid interruptions. For leaders who feel a need to always be readily available to everyone, this can be a challenge. However, it's important to understand that meetings are important, and that getting them done efficiently will actually make you more available to the needs of others.

To minimize interruptions, let others know when the meeting will start and end and when you will be available next. Lock doors (or post a sign on the door) and close blinds if necessary. Tell the receptionist that you are in an important meeting and to please take messages. People should know that your meeting should not be interrupted unless there is a true emergency.

Finally, ask meeting attendees to turn off their phones so that everyone can fully engage.

Doing these three simple things—making sure the purpose of the meeting is clear, clearly defining roles, and avoiding interruptions—will help you hold much more effective and efficient meetings.

Crucial Meetings

Below are the crucial SNF meetings that the administrator should not only attend but should also ensure are being held consistently and effectively.

Daily PPS Meeting

With the new PDPM payment system starting soon, the daily PPS meeting will need to be altered—however a daily skilled meeting of some kind will persist. For now, let's talk about the daily PPS meeting as many aspects of it will probably stay in place with the introduction of PDPM.

The purpose of the daily PPS meeting is twofold. First is to establish good communication across the interdisciplinary team to ensure that all the technical components are met to bill for services provided (i.e. qualifying hospital stays, skilled days remaining, etc.), and that everyone is aware of the potential discharge plan. This meeting includes picking the most advantageous ARD possible that will allow the facility to be paid at the most appropriate level. A review of any additional assessments required, such as change of therapy (COT), or end of therapy (EOT), etc. should also be part of this meeting (these COT, EOT assessments will go away with PDPM).

The second purpose of the PPS meeting is to ensure the facility is doing all it can not to impede the recovery process of the resident. Team members should be asking each other what barriers exist that may be keeping this person from progressing, and then they should help remove those barriers ASAP! It is important to make sure all is done to help the individual receive the highest level of appropriate care so that they can move to the next level of care as quickly and safely as possible.

Weekly Skilled Meeting

The purpose of the weekly skilled meeting is to appropriately verify and document justification for the skilled services the facility is providing. This meeting is similar to the daily PPS meeting, however it includes a more in-depth discussion on the skilled needs of the patient, with an emphasis on good documentation that shows skilled services are needed.

A more in-depth discussion on discharge planning, therapy goals, and PLOFs should also take place during this meeting. Whereas the daily PPS meeting focuses more on the technical components of providing services, such as qualifying stay, skilled days remaining, Medicare certifications, etc., the skilled meeting focuses more on the progress, recovery, and health status of the patient.

Monthly Triple Check

The monthly triple check meeting is a culmination of the daily PPS and weekly skilled meetings. During this meeting, the team does one final review to ensure all "t's" are crossed and "i's" are dotted in order to bill for services provided. If anything is found missing during this process, the team makes plans to rectify it right away so that the facility can proceed with billing.

Weekly Case-Mix Meeting

This meeting should take place in states with case-mix Medicaid payment systems (states that reimburse based on services provided to the resident). In states without case-mix reimbursement, such as California, this meeting is usually not necessary.

The purpose of the weekly case-mix meeting is to have an interdisciplinary review of the long-term care residents— ensuring the facility is doing all it can to help each resident maintain their independence and enjoy the highest quality of life possible. During this meeting, team members should ensure that RUGs are appropriate and that the most advantageous ARDs are selected. A review of all long-term care residents receiving therapy services and restorative services should also take place during this meeting. Whereas the previous three meetings focused on short-term residents, this meeting is all about your long-term patient population.

Daily Stand-Up

The purpose of the daily stand-up meeting is to make sure everyone is on the same page and that good communication is happening across departments. Often, a few key metrics are reviewed in this meeting. The focus should be on important updates that everyone needs to know about, such as new admissions, discharges, pending admissions, and room changes. This meeting should be short and sweet and should not include "storytelling" or items that can be handled with a discussion between two individuals (i.e. deciding on what new dishwasher to purchase).

This meeting often begins with a non-clinical portion that includes all department head leaders. Then, non-clinical leaders are excused, and the meeting proceeds to a clinical portion.

During the clinical portion, changes of conditions and incidents and accidents are discussed along with other important clinical topics, such as any re-hospitalizations that may have transpired.

The stand-up meeting also allows you as the administrator to set a positive tone for each day and focus your team on the most important tasks at hand. It also helps ensure that you are in the know on all important happenings at the facility over the previous 24 hours. When done right, the daily stand-up can be an invaluable opportunity to create the right culture among your leadership team.

Weekly Standard of Care

The purpose of the weekly standard of care (SOC) meeting is to review all the key clinical systems and to make plans to improve care where necessary. During the SOC meeting, in-depth discussions take place on care, outcomes, and plans to improve. Each resident who is not meeting QM thresholds or is triggering for a QM is reviewed, and plans are made to boost the level of care when possible.

Attending this meeting helps the administrator gain important insight and knowledge about each resident. This is invaluable, as family members, physicians, and regulators often ask the administrator questions about residents' status and care. It can become apparent pretty quickly if an administrator is attending the clinical meetings in the facility by asking a few questions about the clinical status of residents.

Monthly QAPI

In essence, the QAPI meeting is a culmination of the clinical portion of the daily stand-up and SOC meetings. Included in this meeting is the medical director, who can also provide input and ideas on improving care and meeting the needs of residents who are triggering in each clinical area. Improvement plans are made during this meeting, and measurements are set to evaluate the plans' effectiveness. When done right, a good QAPI meeting can really enhance a facility's clinical outcomes.

As a reminder, per regulations, this meeting must take place at least quarterly and must be attended by the medical director, DON, and at least three others. Meeting attendance must be documented along with meeting minutes or notes. The QAPI meeting should also be open to all staff and others who wish to attend and provide input.

Monthly All-Staff Meetings

The all-staff meeting is the one (or two) time(s) each month when the leaders of the facility can address the entire team at once. Taking advantage of this opportunity by communicating a well-thought-out and meaningful message each month goes a long way in setting the right tone and culture at your facility. If this meeting is run poorly, it will be hard to get staff to attend, but when run well, staff will be there.

This meeting is an ideal time to provide impactful education to your staff members and also keep them up-to-date on how the facility is performing. Additionally, the meeting can be a great opportunity to recognize staff, share appreciation, and celebrate any accomplishments achieved during the month.

This meeting normally takes place on a pay day.

Consistent and effective meetings go a long way toward making or breaking a facility's results. Note that the meetings discussed in this chapter are not the only meetings that take place in a SNF. There are many other important meetings, such as care plan meetings, for example. The meetings described in this chapter are the critical ones that the administrator must attend and oversee to ensure they are run consistently and effectively.

KEY TAKEAWAYS

- When it comes to meetings, an administrator's attendance and attitude is extremely important and impacts the attitude of the rest of the team.
- Consistent and effective meetings can go a long way in establishing the right culture and helping you run a successful facility.

TASKS TO EXPAND YOUR LEARNING

- ☐ Write down in your own words the purpose of each crucial meeting. Then write down the administrator's role in each meeting.
- ☐ Lead each meeting described in this chapter at least once. Explain the purpose of the meeting at the beginning of each meeting.
- ☐ Rate the current effectiveness of each of the facility's crucial meetings on a scale of 1-10. Then get others involved and make plans to improve them to a 10.

CHAPTER 26

Contracts and Vendors

Introduction

Often, administrators discredit the value high-quality vendors can add to their facility. The right contracts can help save the facility a ton of money, and good service and dependability from vendors can help you meet the needs of those you serve.

Contracts

Many contracts automatically renew each year with increases in pricing. If you aren't reviewing your contracts consistently and renegotiating when appropriate, you are probably unknowingly spending more money than needed. One facility I worked with hadn't reviewed vendor contracts in several years. When a new administrator arrived, he noticed this, began to shop around, and eventually saved the facility tens of thousands of dollars a month. Reviewing all contracts on an annual basis to evaluate pricing and terms can save your facility a lot of money.

Once you know you've found the best potential vendor with the best price, it is important to have your company's contract team review the contract before signing it. It isn't uncommon for vendors to present contracts that are overly burdensome to cancel or that have incremental pricing increases or other terms you may not like. Sometimes vendors may even put a different price in the contract than the one you agreed upon. Having someone else read through the contract can save you from signing something you may regret later.

Whenever possible, request that the contract be for a specified amount of time (ideally a year) without auto-renewal. If the contract does auto-renew, request being able to give 30-day notice of termination without cause, although some vendors will require that you guarantee business with them for at least a year before the 30-day out clause without reasonable cause goes in to effect. Thought not the best case scenario, if pricing is right, facilities can usually survive mediocre service for a year and then change if needed.

Many vendors want contracts that are initially set for 3-5 years in length. This can be risky. When considering a longer contract, be sure to review the termination clause carefully to determine if you will be able to switch vendors before the terms are met if you are unhappy. Some contracts require a 60-, 90-, or 120-day notice before termination of the contract. Others require a documented and justified reason why the facility is cancelling the contract early, as well as opportunities for the vendor to remedy any issues. Cancelling a contract may result in having to pay out the life of the contract—so make sure you review the terms carefully.

To review: ideal contracts are one year in length and include a 30-day notice of termination without cause. This is what you should always shoot for. If a vendor believes in their product and services, they shouldn't be worried about losing your business.

Vendor Relations

Good relationships with vendors can help the facility more than you might think. Providing good customer service and treating vendors as you would treat any customer who walks through your door is a good strategy.

Vendors often know a lot of people and can help spread both good and bad feedback about your facility. Vendors can have relationships with people who you might like to recruit to work with you such as area physicians or DONs.

Vendors may also provide free samples, allow you to try new equipment, help sponsor fundraisers or staff parties, provide staff training and educational opportunities, get involved in resolving issues with family members or others, and make referrals to your facility. The list could go on and on so treat your vendors well.

Though you should always be reviewing contracts and consistently shopping around for the best pricing, keep in mind that good vendors can be hard to find. Changing and moving away from a trusted vendor to save some money may not always be worth it. It is important to ensure that you compare apples to apples in terms of pricing and service and take into consideration all the value a vendor may add to the facility.

Contracts and Regulatory

From a regulatory standpoint, certain contracts are required by law. During the annual survey and often during other visits, surveyors will ask to see certain contracts, such as a transfer agreement or dialysis contracts. This is another reason why facility contracts should be updated and reviewed on an annual basis.

When sharing private health information with vendors, HIPAA clauses and other notices should be included in contracts to minimize the facility's risk and to hold the vendor responsible for keeping patient information private. This is very important and is something surveyors will look for in your contracts.

Having the wrong contracts and vendor relationships can really hurt your facility. The opposite is true as well. Improving contracts and vendor relationships is another lever administrators can pull to elevate the facility's financial performance and enhance the services offered to their customers.

KEY TAKEAWAYS

- Many facilities pay a lot more than they should for goods and services because they fail to review contracts on a consistent basis.
- Good vendor relationships can benefit your facility in more ways than you might imagine.

TASKS TO EXPAND YOUR LEARNING

☐ Review the contracts binder and organize and update it if necessary. If there are any missing contracts, request a copy of them from the vendor. If there are any contracts older than a year or two, consider updating them.

☐ Review a few HIPAA clauses in your contracts. Make sure each contract has one.

☐ Review the terms and termination clauses of some of your vendor contracts. Look at how often the contract renews, how often pricing is subject to change, and how the facility can terminate the contract if needed.

☐ Ask several staff members and department heads who their favorite vendor is and why. Share appreciation with those vendors that receive the most favorable feedback from you staff. Let them know what you discovered about why they are so well-liked by your team and encourage them to continue to provide great service.

☐ Select a contract that has not been recently updated or renegotiated. Contact several potential vendors who provide the same goods or services, compare pricing, and negotiate a new contract for the facility.

CHAPTER 27

Marketing

Introduction

Marketing is promoting and selling your facility to referral sources, patients, families, physicians, and the community. It includes building your reputation and brand and establishing strategic relationships that will grow your census. The goal of marketing efforts is to build census, both short-term and long-term. Marketing is a critical function for any SNF because competition can be fierce and new admissions are the lifeblood of every facility.

Because marketing is so important, an administrator must take time out of their busy schedule to assume an active role in it. Some suggest that 20-25% of an administrator's time should be focused on marketing efforts. This may seem like a lot, but many of the most successful administrators spend at least this amount of time on marketing efforts. Even if marketing is not your specialty, you should still make time to participate in marketing activities each month.

The director of marketing is one of the most important leaders at your facility. Their primary responsibility is to generate business. A good marketer tends to be someone who is an expert at meeting new people and building strong relationships. They are typically well-liked, easy to work with, have great customer service skills, and they know how to sell. Often, they have strong, established connections in the community. To most of the outside world, your director of marketing is the face of the facility.

SNF marketing has changed over the years from simply providing lunches and handing out cookies, facility pens, and brochures to providing real data on key metrics and quality outcomes. Now more than ever, case managers and physicians want to see numbers that speak to the facility's performance and quality of care. More and more customers are holding referral sources accountable for the SNF they end up in and the care they receive there. Thus, great outcomes plus specific strategies and plans to improve your facility's level of performance will help sell it better than sweet treats and an occasional free meal.

Administrator Involvement

As I mentioned earlier, it is important for an administrator to be involved in their facility's marketing efforts. One of the biggest mistakes administrators often make with marketing is relying solely on their director of marketing to build relationships and communicate with referral sources. When this happens, the facility will be left with few such connections if the director of marketing leaves. This circumstance can negatively affect a facility's census stability. The problem can be avoided with ample administrator involvement and having a strong set of marketing systems in place.

There are many easy ways for the administrator to get involved in marketing efforts. A few examples include visiting facility residents when they are admitted to the hospital or writing thank-you notes to referral sources for referrals made to the facility.

Asking for feedback from referral sources on their perception of the facility is another easy way to make contacts, build a relationship, and show your interest in improvement and in meeting their needs. Some administrators even send out monthly updates or summaries to referral sources that highlight clinical outcomes and trends, provide testimonials, and share recent success stories or news of improvements at the facility.

Another way an administrator can and should be involved in marketing efforts is by working closely with their director of marketing. A regular one-on-one meeting is a must. These meetings provide an opportunity for you—as two critical leaders—to discuss the facility's strategies and marketing efforts. It is also a good idea to discuss at these meetings how the administrator can become more involved in marketing efforts.

Finally, there are several simple marketing systems that can be put in to place to help you target and customize your marketing efforts. These include tracking the most recent dates of contact with referral sources, the number of referrals received from each referral source, and logging key information about the referral sources.

Potential Referral Sources

A SNF can receive referrals from many sources. The most obvious, of course, are local hospitals. However, in order to grow its census, there are plenty of other referral sources a SNF should strive to develop relationships with. These include physicians (including specialists such as neurologists, orthopedists, and wound care doctors), home health agencies, hospice companies, assisted living facilities, long-term acute care facilities (LTACs), rehabilitation hospitals, behavioral hospitals, ERs, senior housing communities, senior clinics, and other SNFs.

Let's explore that last one for a moment. If your facility provides niche services, such as bariatric care or a secure unit for people with Alzheimer's, other SNFs that do not provide such services will look to send patients with those needs to buildings that can handle their care. Likewise, some SNFs may not accept certain payer types such as Medicaid or Medicaid-pending, or certain insurances such as Humana or BCBS, so they may look to place residents who have these payer types in facilities that can accept them. For some facilities, marketing to other SNFs in their area produces a lot of referrals.

SNFs that limit their reach and relationship-building to only one or two local hospitals and a small handful of physicians may find their admissions running dry from time to time. Casting a wider net and establishing a good rapport and reputation with all potential referral sources in your greater area is a very good idea.

Growing Census

Besides broadening your list of potential referral sources and building strong relationships with them, there are plenty of other ways to help grow census. Let's take a look at a few.

First, establishing a good marketing plan is helpful, especially for new administrators and/or new directors of marketing who have recently joined a facility. A good marketing plan consists of both short- and long-term marketing goals, along with specific actions and plans to improve census, build strategic relationships, and strengthen the facility's reputation and brand. A marketing plan helps establish priorities and improve focus on efforts that will have the biggest impact on success. It is a good idea to review and update the facility's marketing plan on a regular basis with your director of marketing.

Next, getting involved in the community can be a great way to build awareness and grow your facility's reputation and brand. Participating in health-related community events (e.g. Alzheimer's walks, heart walks, and cancer awareness activities) shows that your facility cares about the community and is an active part of it. Often hospital representatives, physicians, case managers, and families and individuals who could benefit from your services attend these events. You can also offer fun activities at the facility, such as holiday celebrations or community appreciation events. These activities can build awareness and invite the community to come see your building.

Finally, remember to include others in the marketing efforts of your facility. Building census should be everyone's responsibility. Don't forget to emphasize this at all-staff and stand-up meetings. Likewise, some of your department heads may have special connections with physicians or case managers in the area. You might also be surprised by how often staff members have loved ones who need your services. Your DON and DOR should also actively participate in marketing efforts from time to time, as they can be a powerful force in building confidence in the care provided at your facility.

Be creative in finding ways to make your facility stand out and become the facility of choice in your area.

Budgets, Ethics, and Metrics

There are a few marketing budgets to consider and review often with your director of marketing. First is the facility's advertising budget. Different means of advertising should be tried and tested to see what works in your community. Unless a specific method of advertising proves effective, try to avoid long advertising contracts that obligate you to advertise one certain way for an extended period of time.

The next budget is the marketing collateral budget. This includes facility brochures, pamphlets, pens, notepads, etc. Handing out these items and making them readily available to case managers, physicians, and other potential referral sources is a common method to keep your facility on their minds. Occasional freebies (such as hand sanitizers) can help advertise your facility, but be careful to not waste money on items that will just end up thrown in the trash.

The final marketing budget to consider is the traditional budget for gifts, goodies, food, etc. Knowing what your referral sources love enables you to spend money on treats you know they will actually enjoy and appreciate. Providing an extra level of thoughtfulness in gift-giving may help your facility stand out.

There definitely are some things to be aware of when giving gifts. Facilities should never pay anyone directly for referrals. This is an illegal and unethical practice that can get you and the facility in a lot of trouble. And payment isn't limited just to cash. Extravagant gifts, memberships, and high-dollar gift cards can also be construed as payment for referrals. Stay far away from enticing referral sources with what may be deemed as kickbacks.

Lastly, there are several important metrics that the marketing department should track and report on, such as the number of referrals from each referral source, the number of admissions from each referral source, and the conversion rate of all the referrals received in a month. Tracking this information will help you understand where your patients are coming from, where you are having success, and where you can improve. This can help you and the team strategize and develop more effective marketing plans to grow census.

KEY TAKEAWAYS

- The director of marketing is a key leader in the facility and should work closely with the administrator to ensure success in marketing efforts.
- The administrator must take an active role in marketing and help others understand their role in promoting the facility.
- New admissions are the lifeblood of every facility.

TASKS TO EXPAND YOUR LEARNING

- ☐ Work extra closely with the director of marketing for an entire week. Together, establish census goals for the week related to contacts, new referrals, new admissions, and end-of-week census. Visit hospitals, physicians' offices, and other referral sources. Meet potential new admissions and practice your pitch to sell the facility. Close the deal on as many admissions as possible.
- ☐ Work with the director of marketing to identify and establish a new strategic relationship. This may be with a physician, hospital, case manager, ACO, or other potential referral source that isn't currently providing referrals to the facility.
- ☐ Review the marketing plan and help update it if necessary. If a marketing plan does not exist, work with the director of marketing to create one.
- ☐ Review facility brochures, pamphlets, and other marketing material. Can they be improved? If so, do it.

☐ Write at least two or three thank-you notes each week
   to those who send your facility a referral during the
   week.

COMMON POSITIONS IN THE DEPARTMENT

**Director of marketing (community liaison/director of
community relations/VP of business relations)** – Though
facilities use a wide variety of names for this position, its
primary responsibility is to grow and maintain census. This
person oversees advertising campaigns and manages marketing
budgets. They are responsible for cultivating the facility's
reputation and building relationships, as well as making
frequent contacts with referral sources and potential
customers. They often gather clinical and financial information
at hospitals and other institutions that refer potential
admissions to the facility and help evaluate each referral. They
give tours; answers questions from family members, potential
residents, and case managers; and may help with the
completion of new admission paperwork. They champion
customer service and offer input to make sure the building
always looks great. They also supervise the admissions
coordinator and/or anyone assigned to new admission
responsibilities. (Sometimes the director of marketing serves as
the admissions coordinator.) This leader promotes and sells the
facility to the community and makes sure as many people as
possible are aware of all the great services the facility has to
offer.

CHAPTER 28

Admissions

Introduction

Too often, administrators underestimate the importance of a strong admissions process in supporting and building census. The reality is, because of its impact on the business, the admissions process should be one of a facility's most well-run and efficient systems. As noted in the previous chapter, new admissions are the lifeblood of every facility. Without them, a facility can really struggle.

Many customers form opinions about your facility based on their experience with the admissions process. Thus, your admissions process is your chance to make an outstanding—and lasting—first impression.

There are two very different types of customers who are most heavily impacted by the facility's admissions process: referral sources and new residents/families. In this chapter we will take a look at each of them and learn how to create an amazing admissions experience.

Referral Sources

Let's start by looking at the impact of the admissions process on referral sources. Referral sources are those who may refer a patient to your facility as a potential admission. The most common referral source for SNFs are case managers at hospitals.

The speed at which you respond to a referral source will greatly impact census and the referral source's perception of the facility. Imagine for a moment that you are a case manager. You have a patient who urgently needs to leave your hospital, so you refer the patient to two SNFs. One of those SNFs responds to you in 10 minutes, while the other is first hard to reach and then doesn't get back to you for over five hours. Which SNF will you as the case manager be more likely to refer the next patient to?

Now imagine this is your full-time job. You need to find placements for your patients to discharge to as soon as possible and your evaluated on each additional day someone has to stay at the hospital. This is the reality for a typical case manager who makes referrals to SNFs. Of the two facilities mentioned above, which one are you going to choose to refer to most often?

Since referral sources look to SNFs that are easy to contact and that provide quick responses, one very simple yet important way to improve your facility's admissions process is to make sure someone always answers the phone. Rarely will a case manager call a facility twice for a referral unless a patient or their family is adamant about using that facility, which doesn't happen too often. Giving referrals to your facility must be a quick and easy process.

Once a referral is received, referral sources should be able to count on a quick response from the facility as to whether they will accept the patient or not. This is important because case managers need to know if they will have to refer the patient elsewhere.

However, responding quickly to a referral source with a definitive "yes" or "no" is not as easy as it might sound. Typically, a referral will go through two screening processes (hopefully simultaneously) before the SNF makes a decision. Let's look at each of these processes.

One is a clinical review. From a clinical standpoint, there are many factors to consider when accepting a new patient. Does the staff have the skills and capabilities required to meet the patient's needs? Does the facility have the appropriate equipment and number of staff to care for them? Know that once a facility admits a patient, the expectation from the family, the community, and especially the regulatory entities is that it will meet all of the needs necessary to care for that person. You must understand that you can't just simply send a patient out or quickly find another place for them. For this reason, a review of the clinical documentation must take place to ensure the facility can safely and competently meet the patient's needs and provide great care.

The other screening process is a financial review. From a financial standpoint, the facility first needs to take into consideration whether or not the patient has health care insurance. If they do, the facility must verify the insurance benefits and ensure that they haven't been exhausted or discontinued.

If the patient being referred doesn't have insurance, the facility needs to determine if the person could qualify for benefits or if there are other ways the person could pay for their stay. The facility should also make sure the person doesn't have care needs costing more than the potential reimbursement level, such as excessively expensive medications or equipment. These are all financial questions that must be answered before a "yes" or "no" can be given to a referral source. Without verifying how the person will pay for their stay, a facility can quickly fill up with non-paying customers or customers whose care costs much more than the amount the facility is paid.

With these two important screening processes in mind, the facility's goal should be to answer the clinical and financial questions and give the referral source a definitive answer within 15 minutes or less. How is this short turnaround time achieved? With a very strong admissions process, trained leaders, and staff buy-in and understanding about the importance of urgency when it comes to responding to referrals.

The Admissions Coordinator

At the heart of all of this is the person you assign to be responsible for the admissions process. For many facilities, this is a dedicated admissions coordinator. For others it may be the director of marketing, a receptionist, or another facility leader.

Whoever it is, this person must be well-trained and understand the importance of getting both clinical and financial questions answered quickly in order to get a response to the referral source as soon as possible. Many facilities have wisely created systems to give this person more responsibility for performing both the clinical and financial screening without involving others—subsequently avoiding bottlenecks and speeding up response time.

Remember that each referral presents a golden opportunity to wow someone who has the potential to send you more business. Consistently providing a higher level of customer service and creating an excellent experience for that referral source is a powerful way to differentiate your facility from the competition and to grow census. As the administrator, one of your goals should be to ensure that your facility develops the reputation of being the most convenient facility in the area to send a referral to.

Residents and Families

The other category of customers who are highly impacted by your admissions process is residents and their families. Many patients admitted to a SNF leave within the first 72 hours of their stay—often because they are dissatisfied with the service they are receiving. One way to combat premature departures is by having an outstanding admissions process.

Transitioning to a SNF can be confusing, scary, and frustrating. Making every effort to ensure that the process is comfortable, easy, and clear will greatly improve your customer experience and the overall first impression people have of your facility.

Your admissions coordinator should be highly trained in customer service, extremely knowledgeable about the facility, and able to answer or quickly find the answers to the many questions family members and new residents will inevitably have. The person handling admissions should also be extremely patient and empathetic about the difficulty many customers face in adjusting to what is often a new world for them. Thoroughly explaining the admissions paperwork, what to expect at the facility, the health benefits the customer has by receiving SNF care, and the wonderful service they will receive at the facility are all critical tasks for an admissions coordinator. If it isn't obvious by now, the person in charge of the admissions process plays a vital role at your facility.

A good admissions process can help new customers and families quickly feel at home, while a bad one can skyrocket the likelihood of admissions leaving prematurely. The admissions coordinator, administrator, and other department heads should check in with new admissions frequently during their first few days at the facility to ensure that things are going well, resolve any questions or concerns they may have, and help reassure them that the leaders at the facility care about them and are there to ensure they have a great experience.

Conclusion

Your facility's admissions process is extremely important to your business. Constantly evaluating and improving this process is always time well-spent. The admissions process is a system every administrator needs to keep a close eye on with a clear understanding of how it can potentially impact results.

KEY TAKEAWAYS

- The admissions process is extremely important and has a big impact on census.
- Your admissions process is often your first chance to wow your customers and create a great first impression.
- Admitting a patient to your facility should be quick and convenient for all those involved, including referral sources, families, and residents.
- A strong leader responsible for the admissions process is a must-have.

TASKS TO EXPAND YOUR LEARNING

- ☐ Be the admissions coordinator for a day. Answer calls, respond to referral sources, verify benefits and get clinical approvals, prepare rooms, give facility tours, answer new admit questions, etc.
- ☐ Review the new admissions packet and paperwork and gain a solid understanding of each document. Complete a new admission packet with a family member or new resident.
- ☐ Imagine you are admitting a loved one to the facility. Take a tour and complete the required paperwork as if you were a customer. Based on your experience, decide how to improve the process so that customers gain a favorable first impression.
- ☐ Interview a few case managers and referral sources in the area. Learn about their job duties and responsibilities. Ask them how they decide who to refer

a patient to. Ask them to describe the traits of SNFs they like working with the best and of those they like working with the least. Ask them how a SNF can become their go-to facility.

COMMON POSITIONS IN THE DEPARTMENT

Admissions coordinator (director) – Oversees the entire admissions process, verifies benefits, gets clinical and financial approvals for new admissions, interacts and responds quickly to referral sources and inquiries about the facility, gives facility tours, and handles all new admission paperwork, ensuring it is completed in a timely manner. Provides great customer service, is always easy to reach, answers family and new admit questions, and helps them have a smooth transition. The admissions coordinator also works closely with the director of marketing and often keeps statistics on referrals and admissions efforts. This person must be able to work with a sense of urgency and should be organized and able to juggle a lot of tasks at the same time, all while maintaining a big smile. The admissions coordinator is often the customer service champion of the facility and provides training to staff on this topic. They ensure rooms and equipment are ready for new admissions upon arrival and help keep an eye on the facility's cleanliness and appearance. Not all facilities have a designated admissions coordinator, in which case these tasks may be assigned to another person in the facility.

CHAPTER 29

Customer Service

Introduction

If you want your SNF to thrive in today's competitive market, providing exceptional customer service must be at the forefront of all you do. In skilled nursing, it is important to remember that you are not creating a product or selling a good—you are providing a service. The experience you create will determine your customers' level of satisfaction. If you hope to do well as an administrator, teaching, training, and holding your team accountable to a high standard of customer service is important.

The Power of Delivering Service

Think of a company you love. It may be a store, a restaurant, or even a company that provides entertainment. Why do you love that company? What is it about them that makes you love them? Maybe it's the wonderful service you receive, the great pricing, the convenience of doing business with them, or the quality of their products. Whatever your reason, more likely than not, at the center of it all is how you feel while doing business with them. It's the good experience they consistently provide.

The same is true for your customers. If you help them feel comfortable, confident, and in control at your facility, they will have a good experience. If you can help them feel safe, secure, cared about, and loved at your facility, they will have a *great* experience.

As an administrator, you can help your team focus on creating excellent experiences for each person who comes through your doors, including residents, family members, staff, physicians, vendors, and members of the community. With exceptional customer service, your facility can be successful regardless if it is old, outdated, off the beaten path, or if it has had a poor reputation in the past. Winning the customer service battle in your market will allow you to compete against other SNFs in your area regardless of the challenges or disadvantages your facility may face.

Basic Principles

There are certain basic principles that can help facility staff provide great customer service. One is to smile. Always. Smiles communicate happiness and create a welcoming environment that puts others at ease. As people enter your building, if everyone is smiling, they will notice.

Another is using a person's name when talking to them. Encourage your staff to pay attention when introducing themselves to someone and to make it a goal to learn their name. This does take practice but is worth the effort. Whenever you or your team members pass by someone at the facility, be sure to make eye contact, smile, and address that individual by name.

Another key customer service principle is to always ask, "Is there anything else I can help you with?" after serving someone. This is especially important when answering call lights. This follow-up question communicates that you care and want to help.

Creating a list of things staff should and shouldn't say in order to provide great customer service is another way to improve it in your facility. Things such as "that's not my job", "we are short staffed today", or "I don't have the time" should never be said. Make both good and bad lists and then share them widely with the staff. Explain why the list is important and the impact it has on the care provided at the facility.

Whenever a customer says "thank you," responding with "it's my pleasure"—or something similar—lets them know they are not a burden and that you enjoy serving them.

Finally, taking great care of your staff and helping them to have a great employee experience will translate into the best customer care and experiences. The importance of first demonstrating great customer service toward your staff and leading by example cannot be overstated.

Consistently following simple, basic customer service principles like these can quickly improve the overall customer experience and move your facility to the top. Do not underestimate what a high level of customer service can do for your facility.

Feedback and Training

Another important way to improve customer service and the customer experience is to frequently ask for feedback from them. Customer satisfaction surveys can give you wonderful insight into how you are performing and what you can do to elevate your level of service. When possible, communicate the results of surveys with your customers and provide information about what you plan to change as a result of their feedback. As you do this, customers will see that you are serious about what they have to say, and you will then get more feedback that you can act on to improve.

Customer service training should happen frequently in every SNF. Customer service should be talked about during the interview process for all employees, and it should be a meaningful part of new employee orientation. It should be reviewed during all-staff meetings and at other times throughout the year. Customer service should be recognized, rewarded, evaluated, and continuously enhanced.

Offering personalized care, getting to know your residents, and catering services to their wishes are all things that will help your facility provide a higher level of service. So, are you ready for the challenge? In what ways will your facility provide outstanding customer service?

KEY TAKEAWAYS

- Providing great customer service should be a big focus of every facility and every administrator.
- Outstanding customer service will help the facility overcome other disadvantages and challenges it may have.
- Customer service should be a frequent topic of training and education, and it should be evaluated and improved often.

TASKS TO EXPAND YOUR LEARNING

- ☐ Focus on modeling great customer service for an entire week (and then continue it from this point forward). Smile, make eye contact, address people by name, ask them if there is anything else you can do for them after helping them with something, and always respond with "my pleasure" after someone expresses appreciation.
- ☐ Look for staff members who are providing great customer service and recognize them for it on the spot.
- ☐ Review the most recent customer satisfaction survey results. Compare them to results from past surveys. Are things improving?
- ☐ Attend the customer service training provided during new employee orientation. Share your thoughts on how to improve it. If customer service training is not being provided, create a training for new employee orientation and consider teaching it yourself.

- ☐ Create and then conduct a customer service training for your next all-staff meeting.
- ☐ Interview 10 residents and/or family members and get their feedback on the level of customer service provided by the facility. Also ask them how they believe customer service could be improved. Based on the feedback, create a customer service improvement plan.
- ☐ Interview 10 staff members and ask them how they provide great customer service. Gather stories of when they felt they really nailed it in terms of giving great service and share those stories in stand-up meetings and at all-staff meetings.

CHAPTER 30

The Basics

Introduction

You did it! Congratulations on making it to the last chapter. Hopefully by now you feel better prepared to achieve success in every aspect in your facility. As you've learned, being an administrator is no small task and carries a tremendous amount of responsibility, but it can also be an extremely rewarding career. Your ability to influence and impact the lives of others for good is tremendous as a SNF administrator.

If you are not feeling overwhelmed, you are a rare exception. Leading a SNF can be intimidating—there is so much to know and do. If you've taken this book seriously, I can assure you that the basic information you've learned will help you. I also have some good news: being a successful administrator and running a successful facility is easier than it seems. If you do certain basic tasks well and consistently, you can have success regardless of everything else that may be going on. I should warn you that these basic tasks are normally not what people love about being an administrator, nor are they the reasons why anyone wanted to become an administrator. But they are the things that can almost guarantee your success. To help, I've broken these tasks into daily, weekly, and monthly lists. I want to reiterate that the leaders who have the discipline to do these tasks well day in and day out are the ones who find success.

Daily

Track labor—Labor tracking has been a point of emphasis in previous chapters and its importance can't be overstated. As mentioned earlier, wages make up the majority of your expenses. If labor is not controlled and monitored daily, it can be difficult to run a successful building. (See Chapters 11 and 22.)

PPS meeting—An effective daily PPS meeting will help protect your revenue and ensure that you are being reimbursed properly for all of the care and services you are providing. (Note that the name of this meeting will most likely change with the implementation of the new PDPM system.) The PPS meeting will also ensure you have all of the technical components in place in order to bill. (See Chapter 25.)

Review changes of condition and incidents and accidents— There is nothing that will slow progress or divert your attention away from the basics more than poor clinical outcomes. You need to be aware of what is going on in your facility and how the residents are doing. You must stay on top of changes that are occurring and work strategically to minimize your facility's risk and provide great care. (See Chapter 16.)

Verify ADL documentation—Because of the impact of ADL care on reimbursement and revenue, it's a good idea to have a daily review to make sure your CNAs are accurately documenting the ADL care they provide during each shift. Accurate documentation will help the facility take credit and get reimbursed for all the care being provided. (See Chapter 13.)

Review re-hospitalizations—A few years ago this wasn't as big of a deal, but with the impact re-hospitalizations now have on revenue and relationships with referrals sources, they must be reviewed and discussed whenever they occur so that the facility can do all it can to minimize and avoid them. (See Chapter 16.)

Daily rounds—Effective rounding can do so much for you as a leader. Not only does it allow you to see the facility and observe the care and customer service being provided, it also helps you get to know your staff, residents, and the residents' family members. Having a presence on the floor and getting a feel for how the facility looks and is operating at any given time will help you become a respected and effective leader.

Weekly

AR review with the BOM—A weekly review of accounts receivable will help you stay on top of your bad debt and avoid bad debt expenses that can ruin the facility's financial performance. (See Chapter 21.)

Spend-down review—Watching over and monitoring expenditures will keep you from surprises in spending at the end of the month and allow you to avoid excessive and unnecessary spending. This simple practice communicates to your department heads that budgets are important, and that they are accountable for carefully monitoring their spending. (See Chapter 22.)

AP review—Bills can get out of hand quickly if not reviewed routinely and often are full of mistakes. If you are not closely looking at invoices each week, you are probably spending a lot more money than you should be. (See Chapter 23.)

Skilled meeting—Similar to the PPS meeting, the skilled meeting helps you stay on top of every rule and regulation so that you can justify the services being provided and bill accordingly. (See Chapter 25.)

Case-mix meeting—This meeting will help you maintain the highest quality of life for your long-term residents and also ensure that your reimbursement is appropriate based on the care being provided. As a reminder, this meeting is only applicable to case-mix states, which is a good majority of them. (See Chapter 25.)

Therapy metrics review—If you don't review therapy metrics consistently, you may be shocked at the results at the end of the month, as it can be easy to forget about the therapy department. Keeping an eye on productivity, cost per minute, and forecasted Part B revenue will help you make sure the therapy department is providing great services. (See Chapter 20.)

Standard of care meeting—Attending the standard of care meeting each week will let you know the outcomes of your clinical care. This meeting will highlight areas in which you need to improve your care. (See Chapter 25.)

Department head one-on-one meetings—Each week you should be spending some one-on-one time with your department heads. These meetings provide a great opportunity to review performance, talk about goals, and establish clear and consistent feedback and communication. They will also help you drive performance and create the right culture in your facility. (See Chapter 2.)

Write 2-3 thank-you notes—This may not be what you expected to do on a weekly basis, but personal thank-you notes from the administrator can mean a lot, especially to the staff at your facility. Recognizing others and sharing appreciation will help you create the right culture at your facility. (See Chapter 2 and 27.)

Monthly

Pharmacy invoice review—After wages, the pharmacy bill is most often the biggest expense at a facility. Facilities should have parameters in place to monitor pharmaceuticals daily. Each month, thoroughly comb through pharmacy invoices to ensure accuracy and to determine where the most dollars are being spent while evaluating opportunities to reduce them. (See Chapter 22.)

Financial document scrubbing—Though accountants do their best to ensure the accuracy of financial documents, it is important for administrators to review them line-by-line and correct any errors. It isn't uncommon for thousands of dollars' worth of unintentional mistakes to be found. (See Chapter 22.)

Marketing visits and strategic relationship-building—An administrator must spend time each month marketing their facility and strengthening its brand and reputation. Neglecting this important responsibility can really hurt a facility in the long run. (See Chapter 28.)

QAPI meeting—This is an important clinical meeting in which plans are made with the medical director to improve clinical care and outcomes. (See Chapter 25.)

Triple check meeting—This is your last opportunity to make sure all of your "i's" are dotted and "t's" are crossed before billing for services provided. Errors that result from not meeting all the rules and regulations can result in significant takebacks and reductions in reimbursement. (See Chapter 25.)

Inspect kitchen and laundry—These are two areas that can be easily forgotten about if not on your radar from time to time. The kitchen and laundry area are always inspected during annual surveys and frequently during other regulatory visits. Remembering to visit these two areas each month will ensure they are being kept clean and are ready for any unexpected visitors. (See Chapters 4 and 6.)

Review maintenance log and systems—Maintenance is another area that can be easily forgotten and can cause you a lot of headaches if not watched over. Reviewing these systems to ensure that you are staying on top of things and you are in compliance is an important best practice. (see Chapter 5.)

New employee orientation—The administrator should take an active role in new employee orientation each month and, at a minimum, share the mission, vision, and values of the facility. This also gives the administrator an opportunity to learn names and personally welcome each new team member. (See Chapter 10.)

All-staff meeting—The administrator should actively participate in all-staff meetings and ensure that they are a great experience for the team. This is the one time you have each month to share a consistent message with your entire team. Don't miss or waste this opportunity. (See Chapter 25.)

There you have it. Consistently doing these basics in an intentional and meaningful way daily, weekly, and monthly will greatly enhance your ability to run a successful facility as an administrator. Don't allow yourself to get distracted by urgent matters that may not be all that important. Make sure to delegate nonessential tasks and have the discipline to complete these vital responsibilities faithfully. By doing this you will discover they will lead you to great performance at your building.

KEY TAKEAWAYS

- Running a successful facility comes down to consistently and effectively performing the basic tasks and actions that lead to success.
- There are many factors that can distract you from doing the basics well. Have the discipline to stay diligent.
- When things seem confusing, challenging, or overwhelming, go back to the basics and make sure you adhere to them religiously.

TASKS TO EXPAND YOUR LEARNING

- ☐ If you haven't already, begin to consistently do all the daily, weekly, and monthly basics that will help you run a successful facility.
- ☐ Make a personal commitment now to always follow through with the basics no matter what comes your way.

Acknowledgements

It's hard to give thanks to the hundreds—perhaps even thousands—of people who have shaped my career and helped me gain an understanding of the skilled nursing and health care industry.

Perhaps more than any other group of people, I need to thank the wonderful staff I worked with at Timberwood Nursing and Rehabilitation. I've never met such an amazing group of inspirational leaders and dedicated and committed team members. What you taught me and continue to teach me is beyond measure.

Likewise, I also need to thank the amazing staff I worked with at Salado Creek Nursing and Rehabilitation Center. This is where I first stepped through the doors and began my career as a licensed nursing home administrator.

I must also thank my good friends and colleagues who reviewed my manuscript and offered suggestions to improve it. Thank-you for being true warriors and champions for skilled nursing. Thank you for your constant example of sacrifice, care, and compassion as well as your invaluable input into this book.

I'd like to thank my family for putting up with the time it took to write this book. Waking up at very early hours in the morning (even while on vacation) before anyone else awoke made me less than my best self. Thanks for putting up with me and thank you for your tireless trust and support.

Specifically, I need to thank my wife who is always supportive and who always adds insights on how to improve my works. Sweetheart, you are the best!

Thank you to my editor, Diane Szulecki. Your keen eye and helpful suggestions made this book so much better. Also, to the cover designers and others who helped in the design and layout of the book.

Finally, as always, I need to thank my God for his endless mercy and grace. I have been blessed by so many wonderful people surrounding me throughout my life and I know that it is ultimately because of You.

A Formula for Success

In Chapter 2 of this book I shared a simple formula for sustainable success in the skilled nursing industry. When administrators create the right culture, it enables them to retain and attract the best talent. Having the best talent will lead to good clinical outcomes. Good clinical outcomes over a period of time will lead to sustained financial success.

Remember, culture → clinical → financial.

Great Workplace Culture = Best Clinical Outcomes = Sustainable Financial Results

For help in creating an exceptional culture within your skilled nursing center or within your organization, please reach out to me at Tim@TheCenterforCompanyCulture.com or visit TheCenterforCompanyCulture.com.

I'd also love to hear from you! Send me an invitation to connect on linkedin.com.

During the corornavirus pandemic, The Center for Company Culture has also created an online course to help leaders learn how to build their own high-peforming company cultures at their own pace and from the comfort and safety of their own home or office. You can learn more at TheCenterforCompanyCulture.thinkific.com.

The Center for Company Culture offers executive coaching, consultation, speaking, and leadership workshops at discounted rates for all senior care providers. Find out more by emailing Tim or visiting TheCenterforCompanyCulture.com.

About the Author

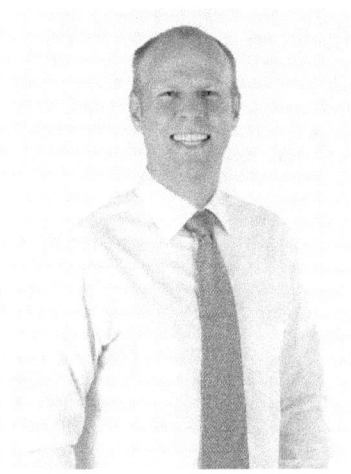

Tim Burningham is an experienced leader in the health care industry, having worked in both acute care hospitals as well as skilled nursing facilities. As a licensed nursing home administrator, Tim led his team and facility to multiple deficiency-free surveys, a 5-star CMS rating, several awards for outstanding performance, and recognition (more than once) as a top 100 Nursing Home by *U.S. News and World Report*. Tim also worked as an area president overseeing multiple SNFs and helped with the administrator-in-training program within his organization.

Tim is also the founder and President of The Center for Company Culture, a management consulting firm specializing in organizational culture, leadership, and team development. Tim's practical and straightforward approach has helped leaders tackle some of their biggest challenges such as employee engagement, leadership, teamwork, and more. To learn more, visit **TheCenterforCompanyCulture.com**.

Tim's other books include *The Wisdom Story: How to Create a High-Performing Culture and Transform Results, Be an Awesome Boss!: The Four C's Model to Leadership Success* and *How Leader's Can Strengthen Their Organization's Culture*. You can find each of his books on Amazon.

Tim lives in the Houston area with his wife and five children.